IN SEARCH OF LONGEVITY

How to Engineer a Life with Healthy Habits

SHELLEY A. MURDOCK

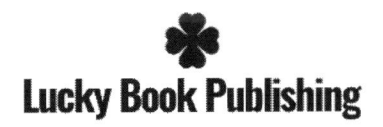

Lucky Book Publishing

Copyright © 2024 Shelley Murdock

Published by Lucky Book Publishing: www.luckybookpublishing.com

All rights reserved. No part of this book may be reproduced or used in any manner without the prior written permission of the copyright owner, except for the use of brief quotations in a book review.

The author does not dispense medical advice or prescribe the use of any technique as a form of treatment for physical, emotional or medical problems without the advice of a physician, either directly or indirectly. The intent of the author is only to offer information of a general true nature to help you in your quest for emotional, physical and spiritual well-being. In the event you use any of the information in this book for yourself, the author and the publisher assume no responsibility for your actions.

To request permissions, contact the publisher at hello@luckybookpublishing.com.

Paperback ISBN: 978-1-998287-61-1
Hardcover ISBN: 978-1-998287-60-4
E-book ISBN: 978-1-998287-59-8

1st edition, February 2025

"Instructions for living a life: Pay attention. Be astonished. Tell about it."

- Mary Oliver

MY GIFT TO YOU

Welcome! I'm thrilled that you're here, embarking on your journey toward a healthier and happier you!

As a special thank you for choosing this book, I'm excited to offer you FREE access to the audiobook of In *Search of Longevity: How to Engineer a Life with Healthy Habits* along with a collection of other valuable resources.

Simply scan the QR code below to claim your gift or visit https://fitnesswithshell.com/

I am also pleased to offer you an exclusive opportunity to join me for an online fitness class. This class is designed to complement the healthy habits you'll learn in this book and support you on your path to longevity.

Thank you for being a part of this journey.

Let's get started on building a healthier, more vibrant life together!

ACKNOWLEDGEMENTS

I would like to express my heartfelt gratitude to everyone who has inspired and supported me on my journey toward longevity and healthy living.

To our beloved Jin-Jan, at 89 years young, who serves as an incredible role model for active and healthy living. Her passion for nature, gardening, yoga, and continuous personal growth shines brightly, bringing joy to all those around her. Your vitality and spirit are truly inspiring.

To my daughter, Bianca, and son-in-law, Adam, and all the busy families striving to raise healthy children in today's world. Your dedication to nurturing the next generation is both admirable and essential. And to my son, Tristan, as a busy entrepreneur opening his first restaurant, he still finds time for daily yoga, which nurtures his mind, body, and spirit. Thank you, my "kid-adults," for reminding me every day of the importance of health, love, and family.

A heartfelt thank you to Samantha and Simar, my esteemed publishers and dear friends. Your invaluable support and guidance have been instrumental throughout this journey. Your encouragement and insights have greatly enriched this book on longevity, and I am deeply grateful for our friendship and partnership.

To my Lovesband, Renzo, who is my everything. Your unwavering support and encouragement have been my greatest strength.

Thank you all for being part of this journey.

"First, it is an intention.
Then a behaviour.
Then a habit.
Then a practice.
Then a second nature.
Then it is simply who you are."

- Brendon Burchard, High Performance Coach

TABLE OF CONTENTS

Manifesto	1
Preface	2
Author's Note - My Why	4
Chapter 1 - Empowered Longevity: The Choices That Shape Our Lifespan	9
Chapter 2 - Cultivating a New Habit: How to Prepare for Transformation	17
Chapter 3 - Letting Go of Unhealthy Habits That Shorten Our Lifespan	32
Chapter 4 - Aging Powerfully Starts Now: Musclespan Matters	42
Chapter 5 - Nourish and Hydrate	67
Chapter 6 - Practice and Cultivate Gratitude	83
Chapter 7 - Neuroplasticity: Get Uncomfortable With New Things and Develop a Growth Mindset	104
Chapter 8 - Let's Get Social: Cultivating Social Belonging	112

Chapter 9 - Alone Zone – Solitude: The Real Self-Care Where Mindset Matters	120
Chapter 10 - Embracing Healthy Daily Habits for a Happier Life	130
Chapter 11 - My 10 Daily Non-Negotiables	165
Chapter 12 - Author's Notes and Longevity Hacks n' Tips	180
Chapter 13 - Embracing Life With My Life Calendar	194
Conclusion - Transform Your Life Today!	197
Resources	198
Meet Shelley A. Murdock	203
My Gift to You	206

MANIFESTO

1. **Live Your Healthiest Life:** The goal is to help you live your healthiest life possible.

2. **Inspire Your Authentic Self:** To discover your true self and find fulfillment while empowering you to reach your highest potential.

3. **Create Lasting Change:** Create opportunities for real change, helping you form healthy habits that are sustainable and can bring you happiness now and in the future.

4. **Influence Your Well-Being:** Learn how you can take charge of your physical, mental, and emotional well-being by building meaningful habits and letting go of unhealthy ones.

5. **Embrace the Aging Process:** The aging process is malleable! Your lifestyle choices can improve or speed up aging, and it's never too late to start exercising and eating better.

PREFACE

Dear Reader,

This is my love letter to you!
Welcome to embracing a healthier future.

Living a healthy life is not just about feeling good today; it is about paving the way for a vibrant tomorrow. Each choice I make today shapes the future I envision for myself. As I embrace my 66th year, I am determined to enjoy every moment with strength and vitality.

I know that by cultivating daily habits that nourish my body and mind, I can enhance my well-being for decades to come. Are you ready to join me on this journey toward a healthier, happier life?

You hold the keys to your wellness journey, and I am here to empower you with simple, easy-to-implement habits that promote longevity. Think of these habits as tools and resources that you can seamlessly incorporate into your daily life, leading you to a deeper sense of well-being.

Remember, this is a collaborative effort. Together, we will build and refine your everyday routine, allowing you to make meaningful changes that align with your longevity goals. It is important to recognize that every small step you take today can lead to significant progress tomorrow—change is not only possible, but achievable.

However, it is crucial to understand that wanting change and actually creating it are two distinct processes. Good habits can easily slip away, while less desirable ones often cling stubbornly. Acknowledging this reality is vital. Setbacks are not failures; they are part of the journey. Embrace them as opportunities for growth. Celebrate even the smallest victories along the way, as these moments of progress are what fuel your motivation and reinforce your commitment to your goals.

Ultimately, your wellness journey is uniquely yours. By focusing on incremental changes and being kind to yourself through the ups and downs, you can cultivate a life filled with health, happiness, and longevity.

AUTHOR'S NOTE - MY WHY

"Age has never bothered me—I celebrate each year around the sun with enthusiasm, and as I write this, I am thrilled to be 65 years young."
- Shelley Murdock

Recently, I came across a social media post that struck me deeply: it suggested that we only have about eighty summers in our lifetime. That thought really resonated with me. As a Canadian, I cherish all four seasons, but summer holds a special place in my heart. Its fleeting nature reminds us to fully embrace and savor every moment. I encourage you to reflect on your own summers and think about how you can make the most of each one. Let's cherish these beautiful seasons together, creating memories and experiences that enrich our lives.

Incorporating daily self-care habits is essential for enhancing your overall wellness and achieving success in your everyday life. A multitude of factors can influence your health, mood, and emotional well-being, all of which play a crucial role in living your best life. By prioritizing self-care, you can create a solid foundation for personal growth and resilience, enabling you to navigate life's challenges with greater ease and positivity.

Do you ever wake up and look in the mirror, feeling fabulous and loving the person staring back at you? If that is you, I am thrilled! But if not, do not worry—you are not alone. Remember, you are the most important person in your life, and you deserve to feel great each day.

What if I told you that it is completely possible to wake up excited for what the day has in store? With just a few simple changes to your daily routine, you can create a healthier, happier, and more fulfilling life. It all starts with small steps that can lead to big transformations.

Imagine transforming your life simply by incorporating a bit of activity into your daily routine. Just a few minutes of movement can elevate your mood, boost your overall well-being, and enhance your quality of life. Picture this: by making healthier food choices, you could enjoy your later years filled with vitality and joy, rather than discomfort and pain. Eating well not only reduces inflammation but also supports gut health, freeing you from the constant worry about your next bowel movement. Instead, you can focus on what truly matters—living life to the fullest and pursuing your passions.

I am excited to embark on this journey with you! Together, we'll explore some key themes throughout this book that can really make a difference in:

- **The Importance of Daily Choices:** Every small decision adds up to create the life you want.

- **Embracing Every Day:** Let's find joy in the little moments and make the most of each day.

- **The Power of Habits:** Discover how building positive habits can transform your routine.

- **Taking Ownership of Your Wellness:** You are in the driver's seat of your health journey, and I am here to support you every step of the way.

This book is more than just a guide to changing your body, losing weight, or running a marathon. It's about embracing a healthier lifestyle that helps you live your best life for as long as possible.

As you start this journey, remember that progress takes time. Every small step you take brings you closer to your goals. Listen to your body, stay committed, and take the time to celebrate your achievements, no matter how small. Together, we will create a stronger, more balanced version of you, ensuring a brighter future ahead.

> *"YOU are the greatest project you'll ever work on. Restart. Reset. Refocus. As many times as you need to, just don't ever give up on yourself."*
> *– Unknown*

Our focus should be to enjoy good health and a better quality of life as we age, rather than simply focusing on living longer. By prioritizing our physical and emotional well-being, we can improve our vitality and overall life experience in our later years.

The goal is to still be physically active and mentally sharp well into our 80s, and 90s, and perhaps beyond.

I cannot wait to dive in and share these insights with you.

xxoo
Shell

"You want to be the person in your family who opens the gigantic COSTCO-sized pickle jar."

- Shelley Murdock

CHAPTER 1
EMPOWERED LONGEVITY: THE CHOICES THAT SHAPE OUR LIFESPAN

"What you water grows."
- The Goddess Rebellion

Did you know that only 20-25% of how long we live is determined by our genes? That means a staggering 75-80% of our lifespan is influenced by our lifestyle choices!

Take a moment to reflect on that.

It's not just about your genetics; it's about the habits and decisions we make throughout our lives that can either enhance or diminish our health as we age.

Recent research highlights that what we eat is one of the most impactful lifestyle changes we can make. By improving our diet, we can significantly boost our healthspan—the period of life spent in good health—and enjoy more quality years as we grow older.

This is empowering news! It means we have control over our health and can actively prevent chronic diseases through better eating habits. The choices we make today don't just affect our present; they shape our future selves as well.

Let's embrace this knowledge and make daily decisions that enhance our well-being for years to come!

Before we get started, let's take a quick moment to define a few key terms. This way, we'll all be on the same page and ready to enjoy this journey together!

LIFESPAN - LONGEVITY

The length of time for which a person or animal lives or a thing functions.

HEALTHSPAN

The length of time we remain healthy and free from disease or age-related disorders.

MUSCLESPAN

If cardio exercise is for a longer life, strength training is for a better life. The term "musclespan," coined by Dr. Gabrielle Lyon, highlights the importance of muscle for health and longevity. She emphasizes that maintaining muscle mass is essential for physical strength, cognitive function, and overall well-being, impacting both body and brain as we age.

HEALTHIER

Improved in health or physical condition. The aim is not to live longer but to age *healthier*, slowing down the onset of age-related diseases such as cancer, Alzheimer's, and arthritis.

> **Question: Why do I use "healthier" instead of "healthiest"?**
>
> "Healthy living" involves making positive choices that improve your physical, mental, and spiritual well-being.
>
> Using "healthier" suggests a focus on progress and sustainability, making it feel achievable for most people. In contrast, "healthiest" implies a strict and potentially unrealistic standard that many might find difficult to maintain.

Take a moment. If you eat a clean diet but need to reach for a protein bar or shake in a pinch that is not the end of the world. Real life needs to meet reality without guilt.

Eating a store-cooked roasted chicken with a salad is far better than selecting fast food. It is still fast food but a better choice. Healthy is achievable and sustainable and guilt-free.

HABIT

An acquired behavior pattern regularly followed until it has become almost involuntary.

ROUTINE

A routine involves a series of behaviors frequently, and intentionally, repeated. Unlike habits, routines are uncomfortable and require a concerted effort.

BEHAVIOR

A behavior must be a regularly performed routine before it can become a habit at all.

GEROSCIENCE: THE SCIENCE OF AGING

Geroscience studies how to slow aging by understanding bodily changes over time. The research focuses on factors that contribute to aging and aims to enhance health and longevity while preventing age-related issues. Although interest in the biology of aging is growing, there's still much to learn in this evolving field.

> *"Health is a state of complete physical, mental, and social well-being and not merely the absence of disease or infirmity."*
> *– World Health Organization (WHO)*

Simply trying to live longer isn't the best goal; I feel it is a misguided approach. What's the value of a long life if the last years are filled with illness, like Alzheimer's?

Our true aim should be health extension, not just life extension. By adopting healthier lifestyles, we can greatly improve our well-being and quality of life as we age.

In the 20th century, we made incredible progress in extending lifespans through better public health, lower infant mortality, and advances against infectious diseases. This shows our resilience and innovation, and now we live longer because of those scientific and medical advances.

> **"What am I passionate about?**
> **Prevention over prescription.**
>
> The real work starts before you ever step or get wheeled into a hospital. This is what I know will help:
>
> 1. Eating well.
> 2. Moving your body.
> 3. Building community/family connections.
> 4. Managing stress.
> 5. Prioritizing sleep.
>
> These are the things we need to talk about more—they're the keys to staying out of my ICU."
>
> - Dr. Kwadwo Kyeremanteng, ICU Doctor

Let's focus on living better, not just longer. Together, we can look forward to a future filled with energy, happiness, and purpose!

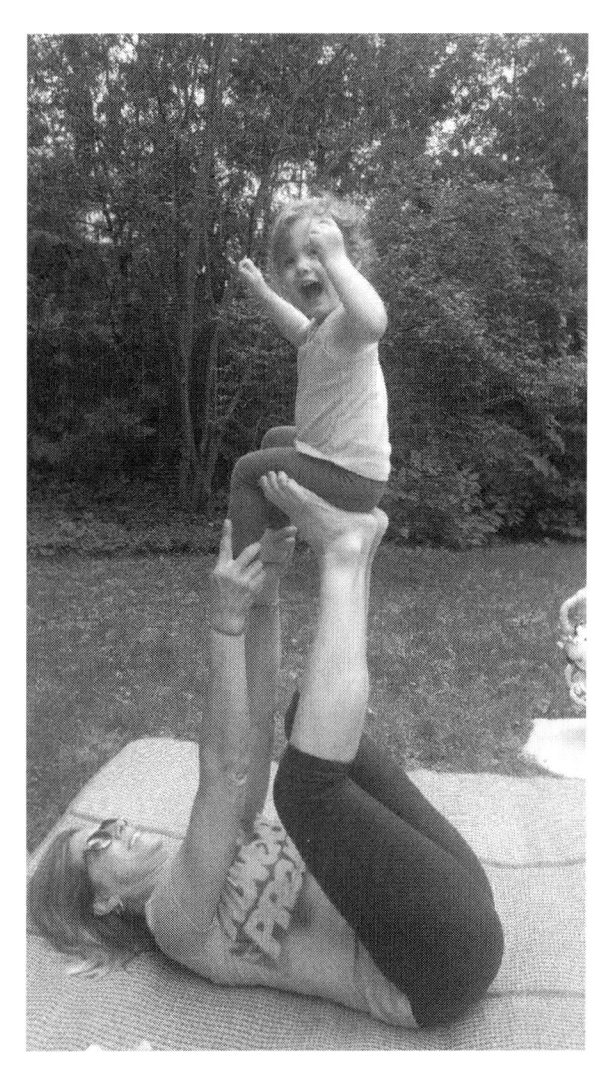

Balance, trust, and endless giggles - pure joy.
Granddaughter Marlowe and Nana time.

"I think in life you should work on yourself until the day you die."

- Serena Williams

CHAPTER 2
CULTIVATING A NEW HABIT
– How to Prepare for Transformation

"You do not just wake up and become the butterfly. Growth is a process."
– Rupi Kaur

How long does it take to build a new habit?

The belief that it takes just 21 days to form a new habit is a myth. While this timeframe is catchy, it can be misleading.

Everyone is unique. What works for one person might not work for another. Habits are complex behaviours influenced by our individual preferences, the specific habit, and the situations we find ourselves in.

- **Individual differences:** What works for one person might not work for another. For example, some people might find it easy to wake up early, while others struggle with it.

- **Nature of the habit:** Some habits are easier to form than others. For example, drinking water is a simple habit, but exercising regularly can be tougher for many people.

- **Context:** The situation or environment around us also affects our habits. If you are in a place where it is easy to snack on junk food, you might do it more often than if you are surrounded by healthy options.

Promoting the 21-day myth may set people up for failure and disappointment. In reality, the time required to establish a habit can vary. Some studies suggest that it can take anywhere from a few weeks to several months to fully integrate a new behavior into our daily lives. For instance, adopting a simple healthy behavior, such as drinking a bottle of water daily, can take anywhere from 18 to 254 days to become a habit.

According to Charles Duhigg, author of The Power of Habit, developing enjoyable habits may require less time, while more challenging behaviors, like committing to a daily workout, typically take longer to establish.

Instead of fixating on arbitrary timelines, it is important to focus on the process of building habits. Prioritize consistency, patience, and self-compassion. Embracing gradual progress, rather than a strict deadline, can lead to a healthier mindset and improve your chances of long-term success.

I reached out to a friend and colleague, Ian Andrew, Group Fitness leader, Master trainer for group fitness instructors, and Personal Trainer to Seniors, for his thoughts on healthy habits, and he shared the following, "As an 86-year-old in the fitness leadership business far in excess of 30 years, one must serve as an example to one's self then to others. No one can honestly say life is easy so I find I must have a positive mindset, retain good dietary and fitness habits continually, and a solid sleep regimen. Accept that which you can't control, setbacks happen. Improve on that which you can and end with a smile even when it is difficult as others could be looking to you for positive support."

Ian's thoughts offer valuable lessons on the importance of mindset, habits, and well-being. This chapter is an invitation for you to keep an open mind about challenges, personal growth, and to be your own ally in your quest to make healthier choices.

A few things to consider about setting a new habit into motion so that you can be successful over the long-term:

1. **Embrace Your Purpose:** Understand your motivation—whether it is a health concern or simply wanting to feel better. The initial enthusiasm is crucial, but keep in mind that motivation can fade quickly.

   Remind yourself, "I am doing this for ME and my future self." Let this mantra be your anchor during challenging times. Practice self-compassion; treat yourself with the same kindness and understanding you would offer to your closest friend. You are your own best ally.

2. **Acknowledge the Journey:** Understand that behavior change is a gradual and often challenging process. Success comes with patience; allow yourself the time needed to grow and evolve. Remember, every step forward, no matter how small, is a step in the right direction.

3. **Pursue Balance for Lasting Happiness:** Our goal is to cultivate a life that is better, happier, and healthier in the long run. Recognize that the habits we've formed over a lifetime won't change overnight. It requires time and dedication to develop new routines that restore balance and enrich our lives. Embrace this journey as a vital investment in your well-being.

Recognizing the need for change can inspire hope, but self-sabotage often sets in before we start. Daily distractions and a multitude of responsibilities derail our intentions, leading us back to old habits and feelings of failure which negatively impacts our health and well-being. This cycle can discourage us from pursuing our goals, as the familiar feels safer than the uncertain path of transformation.

Does the following sound familiar? One of my personal training clients wanted to improve his eating habits, as he found himself relying on takeaway and fast food to manage family meals. Like many busy families, he and his partner were juggling careers, family life, and leisure activities with their children. They often picked up takeaway on their way home from after-school daycare and would "grab something" for lunch.

Determined to make a change, this active family decided they didn't want to continue down this path. They set a goal to increase their fresh food consumption and eliminate fast food altogether. After a smooth start and a few weeks of enjoying healthy snacks and meals, life threw some challenges their way—after-school sports and a work conference disrupted their plans. As a result, they slipped back into their old habits.

However, a month later, they recommitted to their healthy eating plan. This time, they adopted a more moderate approach, allowing themselves some flexibility and forgiveness when life got busy. They realized that balance is key, and they were ready to embrace a healthier lifestyle together.

Take a moment to reflect on the strategies you use to balance everyday demands—are they truly helping you, or are they holding you back?

Here are five compassionate reminders of self-love and forgiveness for your habit transformation–aka your becoming a butterfly. Incorporating these principles into your life can lead to a more balanced and fulfilling experience, enhancing your overall well-being and resilience against challenges.

*To enhance your experience and reinforce positive thinking, consider saying the italicized empowering phrases out loud to yourself. Speaking these words can help internalize their meaning and create a lasting impact. Find a quiet moment, take a deep breath, and repeat the following phrases with intention:

- **Prioritize Daily Habits for Well-Being:** *My daily rituals are the cornerstone of my well-being and self-care. They take precedence in my life. I value my time and ME.*

Daily rituals are essential for maintaining mental, emotional, and physical health. By establishing a routine that includes practices such as meditation, exercise, or journaling, you create a solid foundation for your day.

Prioritizing these habits means they become *non-negotiable parts of your schedule*, helping to build resilience against stress and enhancing your overall quality of life. Consider identifying specific habits that resonate with you and building time each day to engage in them.

- **Set Realistic Expectations and Goals:** *I commit to establishing achievable goals that align with my journey.*

    Setting achievable goals is crucial for personal growth. This involves not only defining what you want to accomplish but also ensuring that these goals are realistic based on your current circumstances and resources.

    Break larger goals into smaller, manageable tasks and celebrate each small victory. This approach helps maintain motivation and provides a clearer pathway to success, making it easier to stay committed to your journey. It takes time.

- **Embrace Progress, Not Perfection:** *I will focus on one small step at a time, recognizing that success is a gradual process. Whether it takes a week, a month, or a lifetime, I am continually evolving.*

  Focusing on progress rather than perfection encourages a healthier mindset. Acknowledge that growth is often a gradual process filled with ups and downs.

  Celebrate your milestones, no matter how small, and understand that every step forward is a step toward your larger goals. Acknowledge the progress you have made like eating healthy foods vs. reaching for the fast-food option or achieving 10,000 steps, and celebrate these victories. This mindset helps reduce anxiety associated with high expectations, keeps you motivated, and allows you to appreciate the journey itself.

- **Accept Life's Interruptions & Personal Accountability:** *While I strive for my personal goals, I acknowledge that life can sometimes intervene. Instead of self-criticism, I will reset and try again.*

  Life is unpredictable, and interruptions are inevitable. Rather than viewing setbacks as failures, reframe them as opportunities for learning and growth. When faced with challenges, practice self-compassion. Acknowledge your feelings, but also remind yourself that it is okay to reset and refocus your efforts. Building resilience involves recognizing that setbacks are part of the process and not the end of your journey. Be honest about setbacks but forgive yourself. Everyone has off days. It is important to get back on track and not let temporary upsets derail your progress. Eye on the prize—YOU—your healthier and happier life.

- **START NOW - Release the Need for Perfection:** *Letting go of perfectionism is key to finding joy in life. If I wait for the "perfect" moment or method, I risk missing out on opportunities. I choose to take action and start now.*

    Perfectionism can hold you back, making it difficult to take action and fully enjoy life. When you let go of the need for everything to be "just right," you open the door to new experiences and opportunities. Remember, it is often better to take imperfect action than to wait forever for the perfect moment. Embrace mistakes as part of the journey; they can teach you valuable lessons and spark creativity. Allow yourself the freedom to explore and grow!

> *"Momentum begets momentum,
> and the best way to start is to start."*
> – Gil Penchina

LONGEVITY TAKEAWAYS

- ✓ Transforming our routines can feel overwhelming and often leads to frustration. By acknowledging these challenges and developing a resilient mindset, we can break free from unhelpful patterns and embrace meaningful changes that promote genuine well-being.

- ✓ When people believe they can easily develop new habits in a short amount of time, they often feel discouraged when they face challenges and setbacks. These difficulties are a normal part of making real changes. This frustration can cause them to give up on their goals completely.

- ✓ Rather than rushing into new behaviors with too much enthusiasm, it's essential to remind ourselves to "take it easy" and approach the process at a comfortable pace. This way, we can make lasting changes without the stress!

- ✓ Remember Ian Andrew's insights on longevity, which emphasized several key principles that can be beneficial for maintaining a healthy and fulfilling life, especially as you age:

1. **Role Modeling:**
   As a leader in fitness, he highlights the importance of being a living example for others. This suggests that maintaining personal health and fitness is crucial not just for oneself, but also for inspiring and guiding others.

2. **Positive Mindset:**
   He underscores the significance of a positive attitude. This mindset can help individuals navigate challenges and maintain motivation over time.

3. **Healthy Habits:**
   Andrew stresses the need for consistent dietary and fitness routines. This reinforces the idea that long-term health is built on daily choices and habits.

4. **Sleep Importance:**
   A solid sleep regimen is vital for overall well-being. Quality sleep can significantly impact physical health, mental clarity, and emotional resilience.

5. **Acceptance of Setbacks:**
   Acknowledging that setbacks are a part of life is important. This perspective encourages resilience and adaptability, reminding us that challenges can be opportunities for growth.

6. **Support for Others:**
   Ending with a smile, even during tough times, highlights the importance of providing support and positivity to those around us. This can create a supportive community and foster connections.

Engaging in conversations about healthy lifestyle habits allows us to share valuable insights. Surrounding ourselves with people who prioritize similar choices positively influences our decisions and leads to better habits. This supportive environment acts as a network of cheerleaders, where everyone encourages each other, making it easier to achieve our goals together.

Remember, your journey can uplift others!

CALL TO ACTION

1. What is your motivation?

2. Start NOW. Do not delay—not Monday, not the New Year, now.

3. How can you improve your life with this new behaviour?

4. What are your expectations on a daily basis to keep this moving forward to a positive change?

5. How do you keep yourself accountable?

6. How do you manage a setback?

7. How do you get back on track?

8. What does success look like?

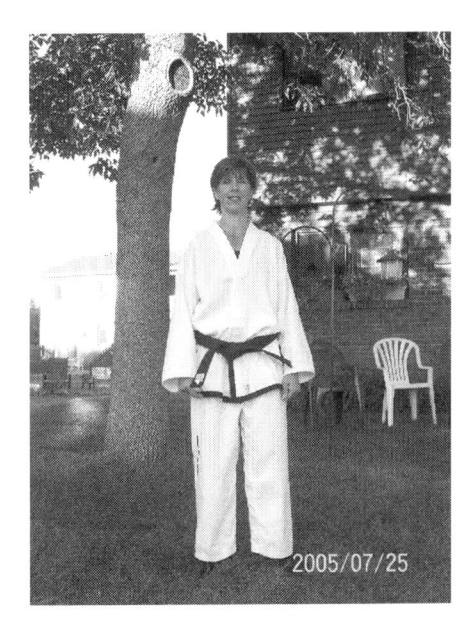

First Dan Black Belt ITF Taekwondo - I love this sport so much. So many wonderful memories of friends of all ages.

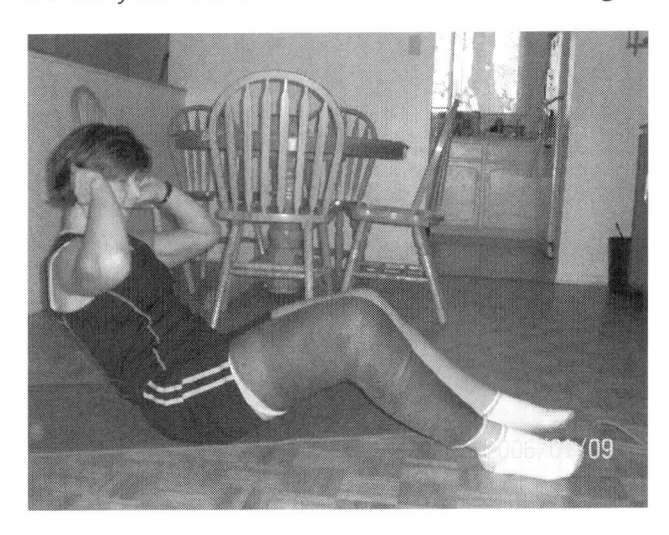

The knee is on a break but I am not.

"In a nutshell, your health, wealth, happiness, fitness, and success depend on your habits."

- **Joanna Jast**

CHAPTER 3
LETTING GO OF UNHEALTHY HABITS THAT SHORTEN OUR LIFESPAN

"Your success and happiness lie in you. Resolve to keep happy, and your joy and you shall form an invincible host against difficulties."
– Helen Keller

Research indicates that a decline in physical activity can begin as early as age seven. Take a moment to consider that: age seven. This highlights the critical importance of instilling healthy habits from a young age.

By adopting good habits yourself, you not only enhance your own health and well-being but also set a positive example for your children and grandchildren. So why wait? There's no better time than NOW to take action!

Become that role model who makes a lasting impression on future generations. You have the power to set the tone for a healthier lifestyle. I find this concept incredibly empowering. It encourages us to take responsibility for our actions and to act as role models for younger generations. This mindset not only guides our individual journeys toward health but also nurtures a shared commitment to well-being. Isn't that truly inspiring?

Imagine the joy of sharing nutritious meals together as a family. Involve your kids in your fitness routines—whether it's a fun workout at home or hitting the gym together. Consider family activities like bike rides, walks, or exploring nature through local hikes during all seasons of the year. These activities not only promote health but also strengthen family bonds.

Instilling positive habits early can help prevent the struggle of making unhealthy choices later in life. Research shows that about 40% of our daily actions are automatic habits we've developed over time that influence our eating, exercise, and even our purchasing behaviors—track your credit card bills for a few months and be astonished or not!

When we think of unhealthy habits, the most common ones that come to mind include poor diet, sedentary lifestyle, lack of sleep, smoking, excessive alcohol consumption, eating disorders, and neglecting mental health. These are significant contributors to poor health.

It is important to also consider some lesser-known and often overlooked habits that can negatively impact our overall well-being. These include inadequate hydration, excessive sugar and salt intake, poor posture, excessive use of devices and social media, and skipping meals.

Awareness of these unhealthy habits is the first step toward making positive changes for better health. Embrace the journey towards healthier living, not just for yourself, but for the generations to come. Being aware of these unhealthy habits is the first step in making positive changes for better health.

Typically, when we try to change unhealthy habits, we often rely on willpower in hopes of quick results. However, this approach can lead to disappointment and frustration, low moods and depression, causing us to revert to old habits. It takes time to rewire our brains for lasting change. Recognizing this can help us be patient and compassionate with ourselves as we work toward our goals.

Breaking bad habits can be tough because of how our brains work. Even if something is not good for us, it can still make us feel happy by releasing a chemical called dopamine. This is the brain's "feel-good" chemical, and it encourages us to keep doing the same thing over time.

For example, let's say that after playing pickleball, you decide to stop at a coffee shop and get a sweet, high-calorie latte and a croissant. Your brain starts to remember this experience, and the next time you play pickleball, you might feel tempted to go back to that coffee shop again. If you keep doing this, it can become a habit.

Understanding this can help us be patient and kind to ourselves as we work toward our goals. Instead of just relying on willpower, we can try to replace that latte and croissant with healthier options, like a smoothie or a piece of fruit. By doing this, we can create new habits that support our health. Remember, every small step counts, and change takes time!

Breaking Bad Habits for Real Change

1. Write down why you want to change.

2. Start making a game plan.

3. Prepare yourself mentally for discomfort and recognize this is a process and will take the time it needs for real change. Think about how you will handle a tempting situation in advance so that you can prepare.

4. Avoid tempting situations e.g. Keep unhealthy foods out of your house.

5. Identify your triggers.

6. Replace unhealthy behaviors with healthier things: e.g. Exercising, doing a fun hobby, or spending time with family.

7. Ask for help and support and talk to friends and family, so they can support you to make better choices.

8. Celebrate small wins to motivate you: treat yourself to something healthy when you reach a small goal. *Recognizing your progress can help keep you motivated!*

LONGEVITY TAKEAWAYS

- ✓ Nurture healthy habits from a young age, especially when it comes to exercise, can have many long-term benefits. When kids are active and exercise regularly, they are more likely to keep doing it as they grow up. This early involvement helps them develop a mindset that values health and well-being.

- ✓ Build and instill positive habits early, as children are influenced by what their parents and caregivers do. If they see their family members making physical activity a priority, they are more likely to follow suit. Play is the best form of exercise, and nothing beats playing outdoors! It's a great way to show kids just how much fun movement and exercise can be, especially when they do it with others. These activities not only keep them active but also help them build important social connections.

✓ This creates a positive cycle in which healthy habits are encouraged at home. By promoting a culture of fitness from a young age, we can help kids become adults who value their health, reducing their chances of lifestyle-related diseases and improving their overall quality of life.

✓ The first rule is to be kind to yourself and practice patience. Trust your abilities, offer yourself encouragement, and don't hesitate to seek help from friends or professionals when needed.

CALL TO ACTION

1. **Visualize Your Goals:**
Picture what you want to achieve and how it will feel in both your body and mind. Make a commitment to your purpose.

2. **Plan Ahead:**
Reflect on how to avoid falling back into unhealthy habits. What strategies can you implement to make better choices?

3. **Identify Your Triggers:**
Recognize the cues that lead you to unhealthy behaviors. Understanding these can help you navigate challenges.

4. **Tackle Challenges Early:**
Complete your most difficult task first thing in the morning when your energy and focus are at their peak. This will help you avoid procrastination and boost your motivation.

5. **Prioritize Nutrition:**
Remember, you can't out-train a poor diet. Quick fixes don't exist; it takes time and effort to replace negative habits with positive ones.

6. **Modify Your Environment:**
Change your surroundings to support your goals. For example, if you want to cut down on sugary sodas, switch to sparkling water. Keep healthy recipes visible on your fridge, and choose a different route to avoid temptations like specialty coffee shops.

7. **Set Yourself Up for Success:**
Make healthy choices easy. If you aim to reduce unhealthy snacking, prepare batches of raw vegetables and have hummus on hand for quick, nutritious options.

8. **Celebrate Small Victories:**
   Acknowledge and celebrate even minor achievements. Recognizing progress helps mitigate the emotional impact of any setbacks. Hold yourself accountable, but don't dwell on mistakes—focus on moving forward.

By using these strategies in your daily life, you can create lasting changes that support long life and well-being.

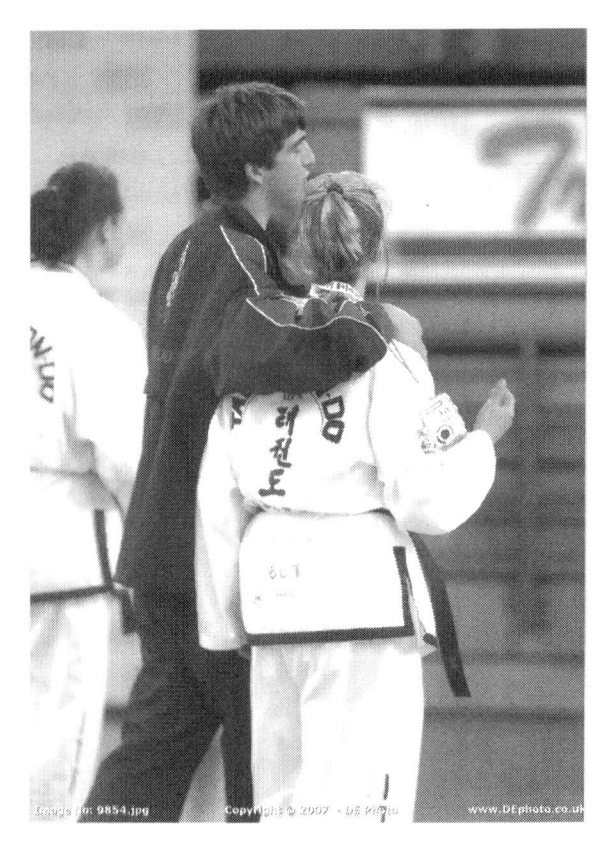

Winning the moment with my son Tristan, who was on the Canadian Boys Taekwondo team, and me waiting for my results.

"The soul grows by subtraction, not addition."

– Henry David Thoreau

CHAPTER 4
AGING POWERFULLY STARTS NOW
Musclespan Matters

"People aren't over-fat. They are under-muscled. Muscle is the organ of longevity."
- Dr. Gabrielle Lyon, author of Forever Strong

We know that aging is a complex biological process marked by gradual changes in our cells and molecular structures. As we age, these changes can lead to various health issues and a decline in our overall functioning. While aging is an inevitable part of life, there are ways to slow down the process and enhance our health as we grow older.

Our goal should be to enjoy a better quality of life as we age, rather than simply focusing on living longer. A key factor in maintaining our quality of life is the health of our bones and muscles. Strong muscles are crucial for everyday activities and help prevent falls as we age, enhancing independence and our quality of life.

Did you know that many health issues we often attribute to aging can actually be prevented or delayed through our lifestyle choices?

For instance, starting at age 40, we lose about 1% of our muscle mass each year, and our strength—our POWER!—declines at a rate of 2-4%. By the time we reach our 50s and 60s, around 11% of both women and men experience sarcopenia, or significant muscle loss. It is surprising that many people are not actively working to prevent this and instead seem resigned to accepting poor health outcomes and invasive procedures. Let's take charge of our health together! Take back our power.

Strength and power are closely connected to skeletal muscle, which is essential for our overall health and longevity. Healthy muscles support our bones and help us maintain balance and stability as we age. During our sessions, I often remind my clients to "hug your muscles to your bones" when we're working on balance and core exercises. This phrase emphasizes the importance of engaging and activating our muscles to support our skeletal structure. By doing so, we not only enhance our strength and stability but also promote better posture and reduce the risk of injury. Remember, strong muscles are the foundation for a healthy, active life!

Why should we care about our skeletal muscle? Our skeletal muscle is responsible for voluntary movements and is attached to our bones, allowing activities like walking and lifting. In contrast, the term "muscle" includes three types: skeletal (voluntary), smooth (involuntary, found in organs), and cardiac (involuntary, found in the heart).

While it's never too late to start strength training, beginning earlier can yield significant benefits. The sooner we commit to building a strong body, the greater the return on investment in our health. This means more years of vitality and fewer years spent in decline.

By making strength training and overall wellness a priority from a young age, we can ensure a healthier future and improve our quality of life as we get older. For instance, the risk of falls increases significantly with age, but we can prepare now by incorporating core strengthening and balance exercises into our fitness routine. Prevention is crucial, and we have the research and knowledge to support this. All we need to do is make these practices part of our daily habits.

> *"If you are >65, and you fall and break your hip, there is a 30-40% chance you will be DEAD in 12 months. This can be stopped."*
> - Dr. Peter Attia

Given we know this information, how do we align it with our busy lives? How do we make movement, specifically strength training part of our everyday healthy habits? Best case scenario is you block time for yourself 30-40 minutes a workout, 3 to 4 times a week. Strength training can be incorporated into your day in small segments throughout the day; if you are unable to commit to a 30-minute workout, then do it in 10-minute segments.

Take a moment to acknowledge that you are committing fully to this process to make it a habit, and then stay present while you do your workout—remember that our habits make us who we are, so it is important to intentionally cultivate good habits.

Unlocking the Secrets to a Healthier Life

When it comes to our well-being, prioritizing fitness is essential. Embrace your time at the gym with confidence—*claim your space in the gym*—as building a strong body not only enhances your physical health but also positively impacts other aspects of your life. Think of the dumbbell as your ally in aging powerfully.

Many people feel uncomfortable and self-conscious when they walk into a gym. With so many different types of equipment and machines, it can be overwhelming. If you have the chance to work with a personal trainer, that's a great option! They can help you understand how to use the equipment properly and teach you the exercises you need.

If you don't usually go to the gym, don't worry! You can start with bodyweight workouts at home. As you get stronger, you can add dumbbells and other equipment. Remember, having a lot of fancy equipment doesn't automatically make you fit. Think about how many friends you know with home gyms full of expensive equipment that ends up collecting dust or being used as a laundry rack! It's all about using what you have and staying active.

It's time to take charge of your fitness journey! You need to take ownership of your workout habits and hold yourself accountable. By doing this, you can improve your life now and set a strong foundation for your future self. Remember, the choices you make today will help you become the healthiest version of yourself tomorrow!

Here are some important tips and ideas to help you create a healthier future:

1. **Prioritize Fitness:**
   Make your well-being a top priority and confidently claim your space in the gym. Building a strong body has massive carryover into other areas of your life.

2. **Boost Your Fitness Journey:**
   Work on improving your fitness and building a healthy body from the inside out. Nutrition plays a big role, so eat well! Also, practice mindfulness and yoga to help your mind and body, and include mobility workouts to keep you flexible and strong.

3. **Healthspan Indicators:**
   Keep track of important signs of health, such as your grip strength and how easily you can get down and stand up repeatedly.

4. **Fundamental Markers of Aging:**
   Be aware of these fundamental markers of aging. By understanding these elements, you can take proactive steps toward maintaining your health and vitality for years to come.

   1. Dynapenia: The loss of muscle strength.
   2. Sarcopenia: The loss of muscle mass.
   3. Decreased Lean Body Mass: The reduction of muscle, bone, and connective tissue.

The Importance of Muscle Health

Maintaining muscle health is essential for longevity and overall well-being. As we age, we naturally lose muscle mass in a process called sarcopenia. This decline can impact our strength, mobility, and quality of life.

However, the good news is that we can take proactive steps to preserve and even enhance our muscle health.

Your Guide to Muscle Health: Key Components

Here are effective strategies to combat muscle loss and keep our muscles strong:

1. Strength Training

Strength training involves exercises that require your muscles to work against resistance, thereby generating force. Incorporating activities such as lifting weights, using resistance bands, or performing bodyweight exercises (like push-ups and squats) into your routine is crucial for building and maintaining muscle mass as you age.

Being fit is essential for living your best life. Before you start lifting weights, it's crucial to condition your body and build healthy movement patterns. If you've experienced injuries, this might also mean reconditioning your body. Our ultimate goals are to cultivate consistency, training more often than we rest, and to get stronger each day, all while living a pain-free life. My clients know that my top priority is to work out safely and focus on preventing injuries.

Remember, your workouts should never feel too easy. When it does, it's time to increase the weight, intensity, or difficulty of your exercises. Workouts should be challenging and rewarding for your body and mind, and besides the exhilarating feeling of finishing a workout you will also feel satisfaction of a job well done.

Here's a personal tip: I love wearing a weighted vest during my daily walks with my dog and even while I'm at home. Sometimes, I wear it while working at my kitchen table—my makeshift home office—where I can enjoy watching the birds at my feeders. I also challenge myself by wearing it when I get up off the floor while playing with my dog. This simple addition makes every movement a little more challenging, which helps boost my muscle strength.

By making strength training a regular part of your routine, you can effectively counteract the effects of sarcopenia and promote a healthier, more active lifestyle. Muscle strength supports bone density, reducing the risk of osteoporosis and fractures through weight-bearing exercises.

From a recent post from Dr. Chris Raynor, MD. Orthopedic Surgeon, Educator and Founder of @humantwopointzero,

Grip Strength Might Just Predict How Long You Will Live

The study states that grip strength can explain an individual's overall strength, upper limb function, bone mineral density, and risk of fractures and falls.

Additionally, there is evidence suggesting a correlation between grip strength and:

- Nutritional deficiencies
- Cognitive function
- Mental health, such as depression and sleep disturbances
- Diabetes
- Presence of multiple health conditions (multimorbidity)
- Overall quality of life

Furthermore, the study suggests that grip strength can predict future health outcomes such as mortality (from all causes and specific diseases), changes in functionality, bone mineral density, risk of fractures, cognitive function, mental health (depression), and potential issues during hospitalization."

2. Protein Intake

Getting enough protein is important for repairing and building muscle. To help your muscles grow and stay healthy, include a variety of protein sources in your meals and snacks.

Protein is a key part of a healthy diet. It's made up of small units called amino acids, which serve as building blocks for your body. Your body uses these amino acids to repair muscles and bones, as well as to create important things like hormones and enzymes. Proteins can also give you energy when you need it.

Here are some great protein sources to consider:

- ✓ Lean meats
- ✓ Fish
- ✓ Lentils
- ✓ Beans
- ✓ Nuts
- ✓ Whey protein
- ✓ Tofu
- ✓ Dairy products

Recent research indicates that a daily protein intake of 1.3 to 1.8 grams per kilogram of body weight may optimize health, particularly in preventing age-related muscle loss (Carbon, J.W., & Pasiakos, S.M., 2019). For reference, this amounts to approximately:

- 88 to 122 grams for women
- 105 to 145 grams for men

In addition, strength training is essential for increasing muscle mass and improving body composition. This process boosts metabolism, enabling more effective fat burning. Pairing a clean diet—rich in natural, whole foods—with a regular resistance training program will help build lean muscle mass.

3. Physical Activity

Maintaining an active lifestyle is essential for muscle engagement and preventing atrophy. Activities such as walking, biking, swimming, gardening, or playing sports can keep your muscles engaged.

You can easily incorporate resistance training into your daily routine. For example, during fitness classes, I like to use workout sliders (or gliders) that slide on surfaces while you step or place your hands on them. This can be likened to tasks such as washing your floors on hands and knees or enthusiastically waxing the car, which adds a fun twist to daily chores.

Remember, it's never too late to start an active lifestyle! Strong muscles contribute to better longevity, mobility, and confidence.

> **Reflections from an Inspiring Practitioner**
>
> At 89 years old, Janet Chappell (our beloved Jin-Jan) shared her remarkable journey with yoga and meditation: "I went to my first class 60 years ago when yoga classes were very rare. I saw an 80-year-old standing on her head, and I was amazed—I thought it was for me. I practiced every day and

enjoyed the philosophy and chanting.

With various groups, I traveled from Montreal to California to meditate at Paramahansa Yogananda's Self-Realization Fellowship, where I sat quietly in beautiful gardens at the retreat. Paramahansa Yogananda is the author of Autobiography of a Yogi. Now, at 89 years old, I still enjoy sitting quietly and doing practices at 2 in the morning."

Jin-Jan's dedication to her practice over the decades is a testament to the transformative power of yoga and meditation. Her story inspires us to embrace our own paths, no matter our age.

3. Adequate Rest

Muscles require time to recover after workouts. Ensuring you get enough rest and quality sleep is crucial for muscle repair and overall health.

The best supplement for building muscle is a good night of sleep. Choose sleep over food, over exercise especially if you are tired. Injuries happen when you are tired.

The Importance of Resistance Training

Numerous studies highlight the benefits of resistance training, including the advantages of carrying heavy weights. For instance, Dr. Peter Attia mentioned in his podcast that women around the age of 40 should aim to carry 75% of their body weight and walk for one minute regularly. This practice not only helps maintain grip strength—an important indicator of longevity—but also contributes to overall health.

My Journey with Farmer's Walks

I recently decided to add Farmer's Walks to my workout routine twice a week, and it has been an amazing experience!

The Farmer's Walk is a challenging exercise that works almost every muscle in your body. It is a functional exercise that involves walking and carrying a heavy weight in each hand, usually kettlebells or dumbbells, for a period of time or for a specific distance.

Within just a month, I saw significant improvements in my strength. As a 65-year-old weighing 135 pounds, I figured that 75% of my body weight is about 100 pounds, and I was excited to challenge myself. Here's how I progressed over five weeks:

- Week 1: I started with two 40-pound dumbbells, completing three one-minute walks.

- Week 2: I added a set with 45-pound dumbbells for one minute.

- Week 3: I progressed to three sets using both 40 and 45-pound dumbbells.

- Week 4: I introduced an additional set using 50-pound dumbbells.

- Week 5: I'm now doing three sets with 40, 45, and 50-pound dumbbells, focusing on improving my form and keeping my shoulders aligned.

Incorporating Farmer's Walks into my routine has been incredibly rewarding. Not only have I gained strength, but I also feel more energized and confident. I encourage everyone to give it a try! It's a simple yet effective exercise that can enhance your overall fitness.

CALL TO ACTION

Join Me on the Journey to Better Health with Farmer's Walks!

Let's lift together and improve our strength! Start with a weight that feels comfortable for you, and progress slowly and steadily. Even if you can only carry a heavier weight for 30 seconds at first, that's a great starting point. You can build on that over time.

Together, we can achieve our fitness goals and enjoy the journey!

Understanding Muscle Fiber Types and Why They Matter

It's important to know about muscle fibers because they play a key role in how our bodies move and perform different activities. There are two main types of muscle fibers in your body:

- Type 1 Fibers: These fibers are great for endurance activities. They help you with things like walking, biking, and running. They support everyday activities such as a leisurely walk or doing yard work.

- Type 2 Fibers: These fibers are all about strength and speed. They power more intense activities, like sprinting or lifting weights.

Together, these muscle fibers prepare your body for quick and powerful movements. Whether you're rushing to the net in pickleball, making a last-minute dash to catch a bus, or catching your toddler before they tumble on the kitchen floor, having both types of muscle fibers helps you stay active and agile.

Understanding these fibers can help you train better and improve your fitness, so you can enjoy all the activities you love!

Ground-to-Standing Exercises

As we get older, simple tasks like rising from the ground can become increasingly challenging. Our muscles and bones may weaken, coordination can decline, and everyday activities can start to feel more daunting. Getting up and down from the ground is a LIFE SKILL that must be maintained and strengthened.

These exercises are important for all of us at any age, but they are crucial for older adults. They help maintain muscle strength, enhance agility, and reduce the risk of falls. Research has shown that sit-and-rise exercises—where individuals repeatedly get up and down from the ground—are valuable indicators of musculoskeletal fitness and overall health. Skeletal muscles comprise 30 to 40% of our total body mass. They are the muscles that connect to your bones and allow you to perform a wide range of daily movements and functions.

CALL TO ACTION

Take a moment to reflect on your ability to sit down and stand up from the ground. Try it out a few times: sit down and then stand back up. Once you feel comfortable, challenge yourself by repeating the exercise a few more times without using your hands.

How did you fare? Consider how you can improve your mobility. Maybe start rising from a chair, or an ottoman or a step stool to start and decrease the height over time.

The Connection Between Strength and Longevity

Research highlights the importance of muscle strength for our overall health. A major study published in June 2022, in *JAMA Network Open* found that weak handgrip strength in midlife is connected to cognitive decline ten years later, according to Harvard Health. This shows that staying strong can help us maintain our mental abilities as we age.

Research published in the *Journal of Alzheimer's Disease* shows that in people with early signs of Alzheimer's, both handgrip strength and walking speed are linked to brain health. Specifically, lower muscle strength and slower walking speeds are associated with smaller sizes in key brain areas, such as the hippocampus, which is crucial for memory and often one of the first areas affected by Alzheimer's disease.

These findings add to the growing evidence that physical fitness is not just a sign of good physical health; they also reflect brain health and longevity. Therefore, focusing on strength training and endurance exercises is essential for supporting both our physical and mental well-being as we grow older.

> **READ THIS AGAIN**
>
> The researchers emphasized that training muscles has indirect benefits that also support brain health, asserting that exercise is one of the most effective strategies for maintaining a healthy body and mind as we age.
>
> Weight training impacts almost every aspect of your life.

Through my years of training, I've learned some valuable lessons:

- ✓ Managing Setbacks: I've learned how to deal with and overcome challenges.

- ✓ Pushing Through Discomfort: I've developed the ability to extend my tolerance and push through tough moments.

- ✓ Building Character: Weight training has taught me perseverance, discipline, and resilience, giving me a deeper respect for my body.

- ✓ Compassion for Others: I've become more compassionate towards others, understanding their struggles better.

- ✓ Body Positivity: I've learned to appreciate my body for all the amazing things it can do. I've eliminated negative self-talk and replaced it with self-encouragement.

- ✓ Showing Up Matters: Even on days when I don't feel like working out, I know that showing up makes a difference in how I feel.

- ✓ Healthy Expectations: I've adjusted my expectations around weight. The numbers on the scale don't define my progress.

- ✓ Body Composition Over Weight: What truly matters is my body composition and overall health, not just my weight.

- ✓ Energy and Endurance: Weight training helps me maintain my energy levels and improve my endurance.

- ✓ Confidence and Strength: I love feeling strong and confident in my body—it's a priceless feeling.

- ✓ Cherishing Moments: I cherish picking up and hugging my granddaughters, and I want to continue doing this for as long as I can.

Weight training has transformed my life in so many ways, and I encourage everyone to embrace it!

LONGEVITY TAKEAWAYS

Maintaining skeletal muscle is crucial as we get older. It helps us stay strong and independent, allowing us to perform daily activities with ease. But that's not all—having strong muscles also supports our metabolic health, which means our bodies can process food and use energy more effectively.

By focusing on activities that build and preserve muscle, we can improve our overall health and increase our chances of living a longer, healthier life. This is important because it allows us to enjoy our lives to the fullest. So let's prioritize muscle health—it really does matter!

Easy everyday actions for a happier, longer life can be easily built into our day:

- You want to be the person in your family who opens the gigantic COSTCO sized pickle jar. Grip strength is related to longevity. Work on your grip strength.

- Weight train, the bottom line is to lift heavy stuff frequently and carry it for at least a minute. Strengthening your muscles boosts your overall health!

- Increasing musculoskeletal fitness through ground to stand drills is one way to build your strength and range of motion and an ideal daily practice.

- By focusing on protein intake, staying active, and allowing for adequate rest, you can significantly improve your muscle health and overall well-being.

- Maintaining muscle strength is important for improving balance, which reduces the risk of falls and injuries. Strong muscles also play a significant role in regulating metabolism and supporting overall physical health, which is essential for a longer, healthier life.

CALLS TO ACTION FOR A HEALTHIER LIFESTYLE

1. Incorporate Weight-Bearing Activities into Your Daily Routine

Think about how you can enhance your daily movements to include more weight-bearing exercises. Look for opportunities to engage in Non-Exercise Activity Thermogenesis (NEAT), which encompasses the energy you expend through spontaneous physical activities that aren't part of structured workouts. Here are some simple ideas:

- Get up and down from the floor while playing with your kids or grandkids.

- Carry grocery bags or heavy items to engage your muscles.

- Reach for overhead compartments when lifting your luggage.

2. Prioritize Nutrition Around Workouts

Focus on maintaining good nutrition before, during, and after your workouts. Consider this: What healthy food habit can you easily implement into your daily routine to enhance your nutrition?

3. Boost Your Grip Strength with Simple Adjustments

Improving your grip strength can be easily integrated into your everyday activities. Here are some practical tips to help you strengthen your grip:

- Use Hand Grippers and Yoga Balls and Wring Out Wet Washcloths: Keep a hand gripper at your desk or in your bag and squeeze it during breaks or while watching TV.

    Incorporate rolling into your day for your hands, through self massage and rolling the yoga ball between your fingers and joints, combined with gripping and releasing tension.

    Use a wet washcloth or similar and wring it out repeatedly. This is an easy go-to.

- Carry Groceries or Heavy Bags: Challenge your grip by carrying groceries or heavy bags with one hand whenever possible.

- Practice Dead Hangs: Find a sturdy bar, such as a pull-up bar, and hang from it for a few seconds to build grip strength.

- Do Farmer's Walks: Grab a pair of heavy objects, like dumbbells or kettlebells, and walk around with them to enhance your grip and overall strength.

By integrating these actions into your daily life, you can significantly improve your physical health and strength.

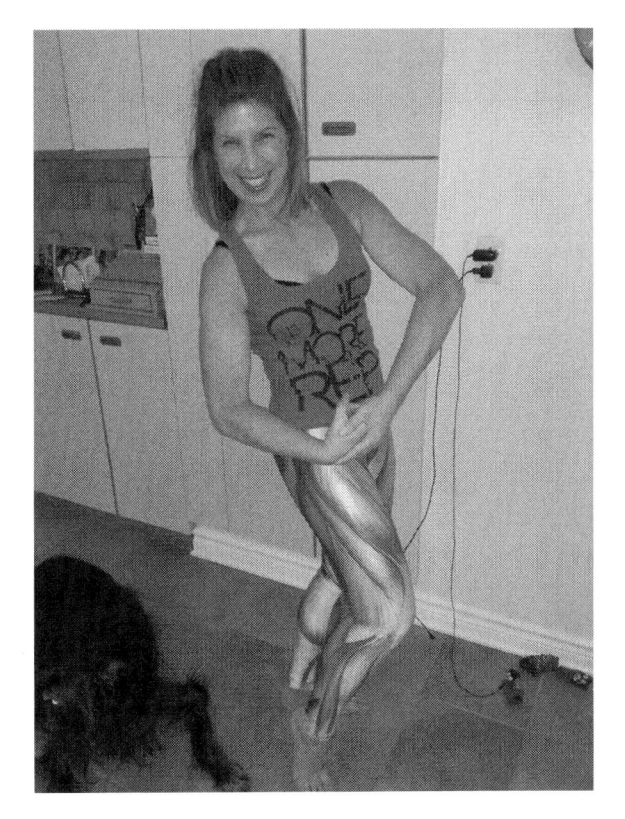

Who needs leg day when you can just wear the pants.

"Remember, aging is a privilege; aging powerfully is a CHOICE. There's no way around it. If you're not choosing to build muscle, you're not going to have the strength to do the activities you love. To prevent yourself from falling and breaking a hip. To be able to do everyday tasks in your own home."

- **JJ Virgin**

CHAPTER 5
NOURISH AND HYDRATE

*"What you eat literally becomes you;
you have a choice in what you are made of."*
- Anonymous

Are your eating habits truly supporting your dreams of a longer, healthier life?

The concept of "rejuvenation" through diet emphasizes how crucial nutrition is for slowing down or even reversing some signs of aging. While aging is a natural part of life, making smart food choices can enhance your cellular health, reduce inflammation, and boost your body's ability to heal itself. This can lead to a more youthful appearance and an overall sense of well-being—feelings of true rejuvenation.

Research shows that our diet is one of the most powerful changes we can make to improve our health and enjoy more fulfilling years as we age.

Eating for longevity may sound complicated, but it can actually be quite simple!

Your Journey to Wellness

A balanced diet rich in whole foods, fruits, vegetables, whole grains, nuts, and lean proteins is crucial for optimum health. We have all read that the Mediterranean diet and other plant-based diets are often associated with longevity, reduced inflammation, and optimum health. The experts tell us, and research shows us that eating nutrient-dense, unadulterated foods (unprocessed) with plenty of vegetables and plants help us to feel better and live better. It improves our gut health (gives us ease and less concern about our digestion and bowels) and decreases inflammation in our joints which causes pain.

Can it be that simple? Apparently yes and no. Why do we struggle with maximizing our wellness with this simple prescription Rx for improved health and wellness? The answer is simple and complex, because our relationship with food is complex and highly emotional, intense, and personal. It is linked to childhood memories, comfort, celebrations, and often convenience and proximity. Habits—the habits we know over the course of our lifetime and what we practice three times a day plus snacks!

Can we get out of our heads and bad habits to eat for our lives like they depend upon it? Because our lives DO depend upon it. The habits of today show up later in our later lives, and with the consumption of so much processed foods, now children and young people are getting age-related diseases. Science backs up that we need to stop eating processed foods—full stop. We are living in an age when obesity rates are climbing faster than ever, and for the first time in decades our life expectancy is declining.

Top Dietary Practices for Longevity and Healthy Eating

To promote longevity through a healthy diet, consider these essential dietary practices that support overall health and well-being:

1. **Eat a Plant-Based Diet**

    Focus on a variety of fruits, vegetables, whole grains, legumes, and nuts. These foods are rich in vitamins, minerals, antioxidants, and fiber, which help protect against chronic diseases. Diets like the Mediterranean are linked to longer lifespans and reduced risks of heart disease, cancer, and diabetes.

2. **Incorporate Healthy Fats**

    Add sources of healthy fats such as avocados, nuts, seeds, and olive oil. Omega-3 fatty acids from fatty fish like salmon promote heart health, reduce inflammation, and support cognitive function as you age.

3. **Reduce Sugar and Processed Foods**

    Minimize added sugars, refined carbohydrates, and highly processed foods. These contribute to chronic inflammation and weight gain, accelerating aging. Aim for flexibility in your choices, focusing on consistency rather than perfection.

    If you can restrict or reduce or eliminate sugar and processed foods completely this would be ideal, but it is not always feasible. Life often requires a bit of flexibility, especially when it comes to our choices around food and exercise. It's important to remember that if healthier options aren't available, it's perfectly okay to indulge in an unhealthy choice now and then. Letting go of guilt in these moments is essential. Embracing this flexibility helps us maintain a balanced relationship with food and exercise, allowing us to enjoy life without the pressure of perfection. Ultimately, being kind to ourselves and recognizing that it's okay to deviate from our ideals is just as important as striving for a healthy lifestyle.

4. **Focus on Antioxidant-Rich Foods**

   Load up on colorful fruits and vegetables, such as berries, spinach, and sweet potatoes, to combat oxidative stress, a significant factor in aging and disease.

5. **Prioritize Fiber**

   Choose fiber-rich foods like whole grains, beans, and vegetables. Fiber aids digestion, regulates blood sugar, and promotes heart health while helping with satiety and reducing cravings.

   Foods like brown rice, quinoa, whole wheat bread, and oats provide essential nutrients and fiber improve digestive health.

6. **Eat Fermented and Probiotic Foods**

   Incorporate yogurt, kefir, sauerkraut, and kimchi to support gut health. A healthy microbiome is linked to improved immunity, digestion, and even mood.

7. **Consume Adequate Protein**

   Include lean sources of protein such as poultry, fish, beans, lentils, and tofu. Protein is essential for maintaining muscle mass, supporting metabolic function, and repairing tissues.

8. **Hydrate Properly**

   Drink plenty of water to stay hydrated, as it is crucial for maintaining cellular function, skin elasticity, and overall metabolic processes. Dehydration can accelerate the aging process.

9. **Limit Red Meat and Avoid Processed Meats**

   Reduce red meat intake and avoid processed meats, which are associated with higher risks of cancer and heart disease; opt for lean meats and plant-based proteins instead.

10. **Seek Professional Guidance**

    Consult a registered dietitian (RD) for personalized nutrition advice. They can help you create a tailored eating plan that meets your specific health needs and goals.

> *"Until you get your nutrition right nothing will change."*
> *Anonymous*

While we can't stop the aging process entirely, adopting these mindful eating habits can lead to a healthier, more vibrant, and youthful appearance. By focusing on these ten dietary principles, you can create a balanced and nutritious eating pattern that supports long-term health.

LONGEVITY TAKEAWAYS

Practical Steps for Healthier Eating Habits

Implementing a balanced and nutritious eating pattern involves gradual changes. Here are some practical steps to get started and make it work for you:

✓ **Plan Your Meals**
Dedicate time each week to create a meal plan that includes a variety of nutritious options.

✓ **Cook at Home**
Preparing meals at home allows you to control ingredients and explore new recipes.

✓ **Practice Portion Control**
Be mindful of serving sizes by using smaller plates and listening to your hunger cues.

✓ **Incorporate Variety**
Aim for a diverse diet rich in antioxidant-rich foods to ensure all necessary nutrients are included.

✓ **Eat Mindfully**

Savor each bite and minimize distractions during meals to enhance your eating experience.

✓ **Shop Smart**

Make a grocery list based on your meal plan and read nutrition labels to choose healthier options.

By gradually incorporating these practices into your daily routine, you can build a healthier lifestyle that promotes longevity and well-being. Remember, every small change counts, so start your journey today by adding just one nutritious food to your meals!

SNACKS AND JUNK FOOD

Breaking away from junk food can be challenging, but with determination and the right strategies, it is achievable. Here are some effective steps to help you reduce and eventually eliminate junk food from your diet so you can continue to build a healthier habit for your body—that beautiful vessel you live in.

Identify Your Triggers and Patterns

Recognize the specific situations, emotions, or habits that lead you to crave junk food. Common triggers might include stress, boredom, or particular social settings.

Acknowledge Emotional Connections

Understand that food often holds profound significance in our lives. It is intertwined with family gatherings, work celebrations, community events, and cultural traditions. These moments can evoke strong emotional responses, which may lead to cravings for comfort foods.

Keep a Journal

Document your cravings and the circumstances surrounding them. This practice can help you pinpoint patterns and develop strategies to manage your triggers effectively. Simply seeing it clearly through the data of your own experiences makes it tangible.

Reflect on Your Environment

Consider how your surroundings influence your eating habits. Certain places or social scenarios can heighten your desire for junk food, making it essential to be mindful of your environment. Consider revamping your cupboards and pantry to eliminate junk food and unhealthy snacks from your home.

By recognizing and understanding your triggers, you can take proactive steps to make healthier choices while still honoring the emotional connections you have with food.

1. **Gradual Reduction**

   Start by gradually reducing your intake of junk food rather than eliminating it all at once. This can make the transition easier and more sustainable.

   Reduce a bowl of "x" to a handful of "x", and a treat is once a week not a daily occurrence. Sadly, we think that muffins are a breakfast food—NO! they are breakfast-cupcakes filled with lots of empty calories, fats and sugar.

2. **Combat Inflammation by eliminating fast food**

   Fast food is often packed with high levels of sodium and unhealthy fats while lacking essential nutrients, contributing to inflammation in the body. By removing these low-nutrition foods from your diet, you not only reduce inflammation but also decrease your cravings and dependency on them.

   These synthetic options leave you feeling unsatisfied and unfulfilled, both physically and mentally. Prioritizing wholesome, nutritious foods will help you feel more energized and content, supporting your overall health and well-being.

Chronic inflammation can lead to various age-related diseases. Embrace anti-inflammatory foods, such as omega-3 fatty acids found in fish and flaxseeds, along with the Mediterranean diet, known for its benefits to longevity.

By focusing on these dietary strategies, you are taking proactive steps toward a healthier, more vibrant life. Remember, every small change counts.

Prioritize quality over quantity; instead of fixating on how much you eat, shift your focus to what you eat. This distinction is key for your overall well-being. Nourishing your body with wholesome, nutrient-dense foods can lead to a healthier gut and improved vitality. In contrast, consuming fast food often results in discomfort and a feeling of illness. By choosing quality ingredients, you can enhance your digestive health and feel more vibrant and energized.

Remember, the right foods can make all the difference in how you feel. Embrace the journey of nourishing your body and watch as you feel more energized, youthful, and alive!

LONGEVITY TAKEAWAYS

✓ *Eating a diet full of ultra-processed foods tends to manipulate your taste buds.* An essential change to improve your nutritional intake is to retrain your tastebuds to eat "real" foods. Eating nutrient-dense foods are filling and you are satiated. It is highly unlikely that you will overeat broccoli or salmon or chicken breast, but the key is to become accustomed to the taste of unadulterated food to the point that your body will crave them vs. the fast fake food (the 3 Fs).

✓ *Fake foods have limited, if not zero, benefits* for you, and the actual manufactured taste is usually chemical, never mind the poor caloric value. Synthetic food leaves you empty—not satiated.

✓ Prioritize Quality Over Quantity: *Focus on what you eat rather than how much.* Choosing nutrient-dense foods promotes a healthier gut and boosts your overall well-being, while fast food can leave you feeling uncomfortable and unwell.

Quality ingredients make a significant difference in how you feel and thrive. Start by incorporating one new healthy fat or energy-boosting food into your meals this week.

LONGEVITY CALLS TO ACTION

> *"We are what we repeatedly eat.
> Healthy eating is not an act, but a habit."*
> — Felicity Luckey

✓ **Review the Government of Canada website, Food Guide, Improving your eating habits** https://food-guide.canada.ca/en/tips-for-healthy-eating/improving-eating-habits/

✓ **Tips for healthy eating** https://food-guide.canada.ca/en/tips-for-healthy-eating/

- Meal planning and cooking

- Planning, buying and cooking healthy food, Canada's food guide plate, recipes, eating on a budget.

✓ **Making healthier choices**

- Diets and Trends: Explore different diets and food trends, including sugar substitutes and the role of physical activity in improving your eating habits.

- Regular Meal Times: Eating at the same times each day helps your body expect food, which can prevent hunger pangs and mood swings.

It also helps you manage your appetite and avoid overeating.

- Aligning with Your Body's Clock: Sticking to regular eating and sleeping schedules is important. Disruptions can lead to weight gain, type 2 diabetes, and heart disease. Keeping a consistent routine supports your overall health.

✓ **Healthy eating anywhere**

- Aim to eat healthy at home, at school, at work, in the community, and at restaurants.

- Limit eating out and look at the menus ahead of time so you know what to order.

- Prepare raw vegetables for quick snacks, add hummus or tzatziki. They are easy to pack for sports, school and work.

- Plan your meals ahead of time so you are not tempted to throw too many ingredients into the recipe unnecessarily.

✓ **Journal what you eat**; make it tangible, make it real. Zero judgement. Then after a few weeks of data, start to improve one aspect each day or week—make it sustainable.

IN SEARCH OF LONGEVITY

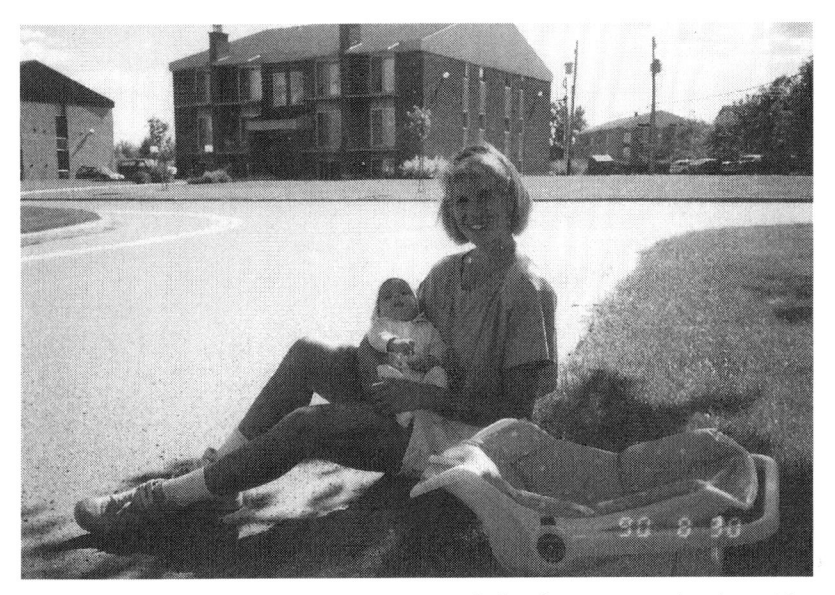

Strong thighs, full arms, and an even fuller heart - motherhood in motion waiting for the school bus for the big kiddo's return.

"Everyone has a doctor in him or her; we just have to help it in its work. The natural healing force within each one of us is the greatest force in getting well. Our food should be our medicine. Our medicine should be our food. But to eat when you are sick, is to feed your sickness."

– Hippocrates

CHAPTER 6
PRACTICE AND CULTIVATE GRATITUDE

*"Gratitude bestows reverence...
changing forever how we experience life and the world."
- John Milton*

Boost your mood with a daily gratitude practice

Gratitude, derived from the Latin word "gratia," means gratefulness or thankfulness. "Gratitude is not only the greatest of virtues, but the parent of all others," according to Marcus Tullius Cicero.

We all crave a happy life. When we think about what brings us joy, we often focus on those big, unforgettable moments—like holidays or special events filled with intense emotions. But interestingly, it's the small, everyday moments that really contribute to our happiness and overall satisfaction.

What brings you joy? Is it spending time with family and friends, volunteering, enjoying music, or dancing? Think about the activities and relationships that shape the way you see the world. Take a moment to reflect on what helps you cultivate a more optimistic outlook on life.

Gratitude is a powerful source of happiness. It enhances our sense of pleasure and well-being, ultimately benefiting our health. By focusing on gratitude and personal growth, we can strengthen our emotional resilience.

Expressing gratitude can improve our relationships—whether at home with family, at work with colleagues, or with friends. Building deeper, lasting connections is essential for a fulfilling and healthy life.

Research shows that practicing gratitude can really help us see the good things in our lives and inspire us to spread that positivity to others. People who focus on gratitude often feel happier and more satisfied with their lives. It also helps us connect with others, forming new friendships and strengthening the ones we already have, which builds a strong community. Additionally, studies suggest that being grateful can positively affect how our brains work.

Gratitude is a relatively new area of study, but it's showing some exciting findings. Research shows that when we practice gratitude, we tend to be kinder and more generous, which helps strengthen our relationships with others. This not only makes our connections deeper but also has lasting benefits for our lives.

Having a grateful mindset can greatly improve our happiness, satisfaction, and optimism. Interestingly, a survey by Robert Holden, a British psychologist and wellness expert, found that 65 out of 100 people would choose happiness over health, even though they acknowledged that both are important for a fulfilling life.

It's easy to feel grateful when everything is going well. But let's be honest—when life throws us a curveball, it can be really hard to find that sense of gratitude. When things go wrong and it feels like everything is falling apart, gratitude is often the last thing on our minds. I remember a funny meme that captures this feeling perfectly, especially on those clumsy days when it seems like nothing is going right. It goes something like this: "Why do I bump my elbow into everything when I'm running late?" It perfectly sums up those frustrating moments!

> *"It is impossible to feel depressed and grateful at the same moment."*
> *– Naomi Williams*

Our brains are naturally wired to pay more attention to negative things, a trait that helped our ancestors survive. However, this tendency can make us jump to negative conclusions or think the worst, which isn't helpful in our current daily lives. Engaging in catastrophic thinking is not helpful. By improving our observation skills and accepting life as it really is, with its ups and downs, we can better tell the difference between real dangers and things we worry about that aren't actually a threat. This helps us appreciate the good things around us more.

> *"Gratitude drives happiness. Happiness boosts productivity. Productivity reveals mastery. And mastery inspires the world."*
> *– Robin Sharma*

Gratitude is a powerful practice that can greatly improve our emotional and psychological well-being. It can enhance our lives in two main ways: by boosting our mental health and possibly even extending our lifespan. Here's how it works:

1. **Enhanced Mental Health**

    ✓ **Promotes Positive Emotions**

    Practicing gratitude helps us feel joy, contentment, and love. These positive feelings can reduce negative emotions like envy and resentment.

    Feeling joy regularly improves our mental health and lowers the risk of depression and anxiety, which are often connected to lower life satisfaction and shorter lifespans.

    ✓ **Builds Resilience**

    Gratitude helps us become more resilient, allowing us to handle stress and challenges better. This resilience is important for mental health, helping us recover from setbacks more quickly. A resilient mindset boosts happiness and may even lead to a longer life.

    ✓ Gratitude builds emotional resilience by:

    - Helping us notice the positive things in life.

    - Reducing negative thoughts and replacing them with positive ones, stopping the negative ruminations and pessimistic thoughts.

- Keeping us grounded and accepting our current situation, even if it's tough.

- Focusing on solutions instead of problems.

- Supporting our health by regulating our body's functions and balancing hormones.

- Strengthening relationships and appreciating the people who support us, making us feel more loved and hopeful.

2. **Improved Physical Health**

- Stress Reduction: Gratitude helps lower stress hormones like cortisol. Reducing stress can protect you from serious health problems, such as heart disease and high blood pressure, leading to a longer, healthier life.

- Healthier Habits: People who focus on gratitude are more likely to exercise, eat well, and get enough sleep. Gratitude also promotes better self-care and helps you stick to medical advice, which boosts overall health.

3. **Stronger Social Connections**

- Building Relationships: Expressing gratitude helps us build trust and respect with others. Strong relationships are important for our mental and physical health. They provide emotional support, reduce loneliness, and increase life satisfaction. There is a significant body of research that indicates that social support is linked to lower rates of chronic disease and better recovery from illness.

- Empathy and Altruism: Gratitude encourages empathy and a desire to help others, which strengthens our relationships and builds a supportive community. Feeling connected to others is essential for our happiness and longevity.

4. **Increased Life Satisfaction and Happiness**

- Mindset Shift: Practicing gratitude helps you focus on what you have instead of what you lack. This shift reduces negative thoughts and promotes a more positive outlook, leading to greater happiness and life satisfaction. A positive mindset is also connected to healthier aging and a longer life.

- Contentment: By appreciating what you have, gratitude promotes a sense of contentment. This reduces the urge to constantly compare yourself to others, resulting in a more peaceful and fulfilling life, which enhances overall happiness.

> *"Feeling gratitude and not expressing it is like wrapping a present and not giving it."*
> *- William Arthur Ward*

5. **Better Sleep Quality**

- Relaxation and Rest: Engaging in gratitude practices, especially before bedtime—like journaling or reflecting on the positive aspects of your day—can improve sleep quality. Better sleep is associated with many health benefits, including enhanced immune function, better mental health, and a lower risk of chronic diseases, all contributing to a longer life.

6. **Lower Risk of Chronic Diseases**

- Cardiovascular Health: Gratitude is linked to better heart health, including lower blood pressure and a reduced risk of heart disease. The positive feelings from gratitude can lower inflammation and improve heart rate, both signs of a healthy cardiovascular system.

- Immune Function: Practicing gratitude can boost your immune system, making you more resistant to illness. A strong immune system is important for a long life, as it helps protect against diseases.

7. Increased Motivation and Goal Achievement

- Focus and Perseverance: Grateful people are often more motivated and persistent in reaching their goals. Gratitude helps them stay focused on their long-term dreams, encouraging actions that lead to personal fulfillment and well-being. Accomplishing meaningful goals can enhance life satisfaction and gives a sense of purpose, which can contribute to a longer life.

8. Encourages a Sense of Purpose

- Meaning in Life: Gratitude often deepens your appreciation for life's experiences, building a stronger sense of purpose and meaning. Having a sense of purpose has been shown to positively impact health and longevity, encouraging active engagement in life and the pursuit of meaningful activities.

  Finding activities that bring you joy, and a sense of purpose is important for feeling connected and accomplished, as everyone is unique. You might invest time in friendships and relationships to build deeper connections or volunteer in your community to find fulfillment by helping others. Additionally, pursuing hobbies and passions such as painting or gardening can provide an outlet for your creativity. These simple actions can greatly enhance your happiness and sense of purpose.

> *"Give yourself a gift of five minutes of contemplation in awe of everything you see around you. Go outside and turn your attention to the many miracles around you. This five-minute-a-day regimen of appreciation and gratitude will help you to focus your life in awe."*
> – Wayne Dyer

Gratitude is a powerful tool for enhancing happiness and potentially extending lifespan. By improving mental and physical health, fostering strong social connections, and promoting a positive outlook on life, gratitude contributes to a more fulfilling, healthier, and longer life.

FAST FACTS
Why gratitude is an underrated free and powerful medicine.

It may :

- Improve a healthy nervous system regulation.
- Improve your overall happiness.
- Improve anxiety and depression.
- Improve your relationships.

- Improve perspective regarding stress.
- Improve your resilience.
- Improve your self-esteem.
- Improve your living in alignment .
- Improve your quality of sleep.
- Improve your ability to cope with stress.
- Improve focusing on what really matters.
- Improve your outlook/hope for the future.
- Improve your physical and mental well-being.
- Improve the release of serotonin and dopamine.

LONGEVITY GRATITUDE PRACTICES

1. **Express Thanks:** Take a moment to thank someone who has made a positive impact on your life. A simple "thank you" sends a message of encouragement, which builds relationships, and this expression of gratitude induces positive emotions, a sense of contentment for both the giver and the receiver, which impacts our well-being in a positive way.

2. **Marta Zaraska, in her book Growing Young:** How Friendship, Optimism, and Kindness Can Help You Live to 100, emphasizes the profound impact of social connections and kindness on

longevity. She notes, "Yet now I know [socializing while exercising] can be actually more important to my longevity than extra training sessions. I also make sure to do more sports together with other people." This highlights the idea that engaging with others while being active not only enhances our physical health but also strengthens our bonds, contributing significantly to our overall well-being.

Zaraska further illustrates the importance of kindness in our daily lives, stating, "I try to do more acts of kindness; it can be as simple as picking litter on the way to a store or letting others ahead in traffic." These small acts of kindness not only help the people around us but also make us feel good and grateful, which is important for our happiness and health. Together, these ideas show how friendships and being kind can help us live longer and happier lives.

Plogging is the latest trend in fitness; it is the act of picking up litter while you jog or run. It is a great initiative to start in your neighborhood or community; the opportunity to get fit and help the environment is a win-win.

3. **Foster a mindset of gratitude, reflection, and self-care** as you bring your goals and dreams to life. Welcome each morning as a chance to unlock your potential, infusing your day with intention, productivity, and joy.

4. **To enhance your daily routine, consider integrating the STOP mindfulness technique** at a consistent time each day, transforming it into a positive habit. The STOP technique consists of a simple four-step mental checklist designed to help you anchor yourself in the present moment. By regularly practicing this method, you can cultivate mindfulness, reduce stress, and improve your overall well-being. Making this a dedicated part of your day ensures that you take a moment to pause, reflect, and reconnect with yourself, fostering a deeper sense of awareness and tranquility.

   The STOP acronym stands for:
   - ✓ Stop
   - ✓ Take a breath
   - ✓ Observe
   - ✓ Proceed

5. **Reflect:** At the end of each week, reflect on what you appreciated most.

6. **Create a Gratitude Journal aka Your JOY Journal:** Write down three things you're thankful for each day.

Maintaining new habits depend on a few factors to reinforce and encourage behaviour. One of the best ways to stick to your new healthier and happier habit is by tracking it through journaling. Additionally, the actual act of writing by hand has both physical and visual impacts, which allows you to see and monitor your progress. By journaling you are keeping yourself accountable, which is key for maintenance and sustainability.

To encourage you to build a daily habit of a gratitude journal, I invite you to explore the below exercise. The goal is for you to cultivate a deeper sense of gratitude and transform your mindset through consistent practice, making it a healthy habit. Keep in mind that happiness is personal, and the journey towards it should be adaptive to your evolving lifestyle.

- Simply stop, pause to reflect upon your day, and observe without judgement the moments that brought you joy.

- Take the time to discern what will enhance your emotional, mental, and physical well-being daily, and then write them down.

- Please remember this is a personal growth opportunity, as we want to know how to deliberately create positive habits that can be found in everyday activities and that are sustainable.

You may want to implement the STOP mindfulness technique to prepare for your journaling.

YOUR JOY LIST

What activities bring you joy?

Identify three (3) specific activities that bring you pleasure and that you look forward to participating in or experiencing:

1. _____

2. _____

3. _____

DAILY JOURNAL PROMPTS

Today I am grateful for:

1. _____

2. _____

3. _____

One (1) person I am thankful for today:

_____

One (1) challenge I encountered and managed today.

_____

What did I learn from this experience? Look for the lesson to help you move forward.

_____

REFLECTIONS on today, look at the BIG picture and list your thoughts and gifts for tomorrow:

WEEKLY   1. _____

                  2. _____

                  3. _____

MONTHLY 1. _____

                  2. _____

                  3. _____

ANNUALLY 1. _____

2. _____

3. _____

Gratitude Meditation Practice

A morning meditation ritual is a wonderful way to set the tone for your day. It can help you to be prepared to respond in peace and positivity to the events of the day as they unfold so that you can be successful and feel good about your emotional health. Using deep breathing exercises with a continuous focus on your breath will allow your mind to slow down and give you a deeper connection to yourself.

Here is a 2-minute meditation session that you can follow:

1. Begin by finding a comfortable and stable seat where the spine is long and the chest is broad.

2. Call upon the feeling of ease by bringing a soft smile to the lips and closed eyes.

3. Pay attention to the natural rhythm of the breath.

4. Then mentally express why you are grateful. Do this until the feeling of gratitude permeates your body and mind.

5. Once the feeling flows, give your attention to the feeling. If you lose the feeling, go back to mentally expressing your gratitude.

6. You can do this for as little as 2 minutes to as long as you feel you need.

CALL TO ACTION

Your JOY list – what brings you joy?

1. _____

2. _____

3. _____

4. _____

5. _____

Forming new happiness habits:

Daily

Weekly

Monthly

Annually

LONGEVITY TAKEAWAY

Gratitude has a profound impact to create a happier life and potentially extend lifespan.

Incorporating gratitude into our daily routines helps us retrain our focus on the world around us. By consciously appreciating the positive aspects of our everyday lives while acknowledging the challenges we face, we become more aware and balanced in our experiences.

> *"Foster gratitude into every day."*
> *– The Goddess of Rebellion*

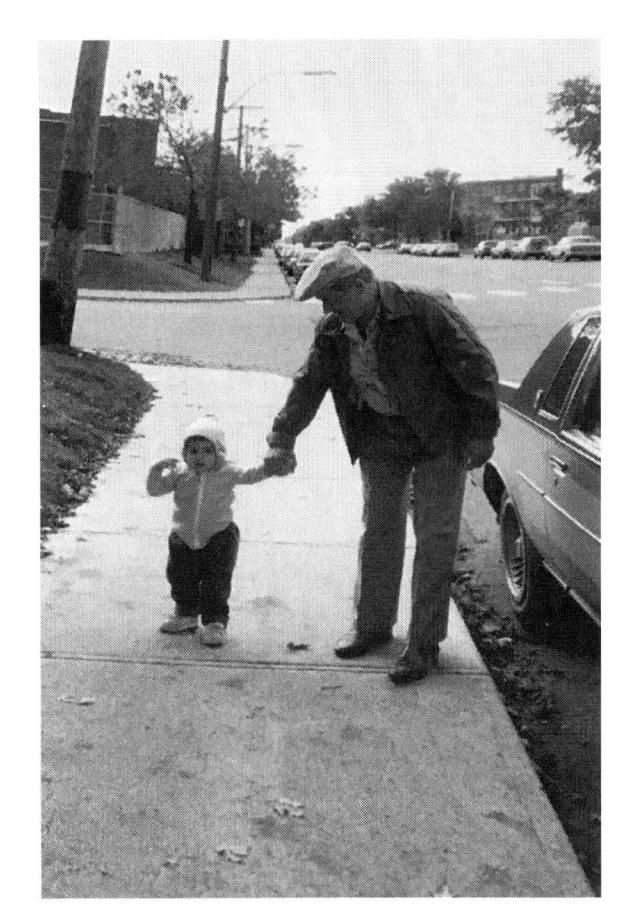

This is my daughter and father-in-law.
Generations connected - love that lasts a lifetime.

"Gratitude is the healthiest of all human emotions. The more you express gratitude for what you have, the more likely you will have even more to express gratitude for."

— Zig Ziglar

CHAPTER 7
NEUROPLASTICITY
Get Uncomfortable with New Things and Develop a Growth Mindset

"If you can change your mind, you can change your life."
– James William

Continuous learning is a vital habit for longevity. If you cease to learn new things, then you are aging! By learning new skills, you are benefiting both your mental and physical well-being, which keeps you active longer and engaged in life.

Neuroplasticity is your brain's ability to learn and adapt to new challenges. Just like your body needs to workout, so does your brain. Brain-building and using the three-pound organ in your head helps it become flexible just like your muscles, so that it can adapt and readjust to new experiences.

Lifelong learning keeps your brain active and helps maintain cognitive function as you age. This can include reading, taking courses, learning new skills, or simply staying curious about life. Continuously exposing your brain to new experiences and activities allows you to make better decisions and solve problems more effectively. Staying engaged and learning throughout life can lead to greater mental sharpness and overall well-being.

- ✓ Reading books and articles keeps your mind engaged and exposes you to new ideas and knowledge.

- ✓ Taking courses, whether in-person or online, can keep your mind sharp, and if you are seeking new skills or topics of interest, there are endless possibilities to keep your brain engaged and challenged.

- ✓ Learning a new skill or picking up a new hobby like playing an instrument, or learning a new language, or even cooking a new recipe can be stimulating.

- ✓ Staying curious and asking questions about the world around you or far away or exploring new topics can be fun and adventurous.

In the article, *Brainwork: The Power of Neuroplasticity*, for Health Essentials from Cleveland Clinic, psychologist Grace Tworek, PsyD made some recommendations to improve your brain power that don't require you making huge life changes. Dr. Tworek shared, "You don't need to travel across the world to find new experiences, instead, look to build the concept of 'new experiences' into your day-to-day life with some simple acts." Read the full article here https://health.clevelandclinic.org/neuroplasticity

Here are some ideas to flex our brain and add some fun to our lives:

- ✓ Try a new exercise routine or new physical activity, i.e. if you are a runner try a sport or do an interval training class.

- ✓ Brain aerobics:
    - Get dressed standing on one leg.
    - Use your non-dominant hand to do everyday activities, like brushing your hair or your teeth, opening doors, etc.

- ✓ Practice remembering people's names.

- ✓ Use different routes to get to places instead of the usual route, and without using your GPS.

- ✓ Expand your vocabulary and learn how to spell and pronounce the word, as auditory learning is as important for memory as visual learning.

- ✓ Use mnemonic strategies – rhyming (like "i" before "e" except after "c"), or number sequencing (chunking numbers out like a phone number, social security number, etc.), or practicing acronyms are useful.

- ✓ Getting enough sleep, rest, and naps. "Sleep is when the information from the day is being consolidated in your brain," says Dr. Tworek. "It helps your brain more than you can imagine."

- ✓ Play video games! Puzzle games, 3D games, Tetris, dance simulators all improve your brain and visuospatial skills e.g. jigsaw puzzles, putting together unassembled furniture. Presently, there is limited research on the long-term effects of video games and memory.

- ✓ Music combined with dance, exercise or gaming promotes neuroplasticity. Music therapy has proven to be successful in strengthening memory ability.

- ✓ Drawing, painting, and creating art can deepen your emotions, give you insights to things that you were not aware of, and help you to connect with yourself and your surroundings, and they can improve your brain function by creating new pathways.

LONGEVITY CALLS TO ACTION

How to get started:

1. Is there something you have always wanted to try or learn? Make a list of five things you have always wanted to do. Which one resonates with you the deepest?

2. Why do you want to learn this skill? What is the attachment to you, what is its importance to you—the intention is key. It could be because you have always wanted to learn to play an instrument.

3. Commit to the challenge. Upper case letters COMMIT. All in and no half-measures.

4. Put a plan in action, and schedule time to practice the skill as frequently as you can through the week to make it fun and challenging, not a chore.

5. Repetition - repetition - REPETITION.

6. Check in with yourself weekly to see whether you are progressing. Be patient and plan for relapses, and just refocus, it takes time.

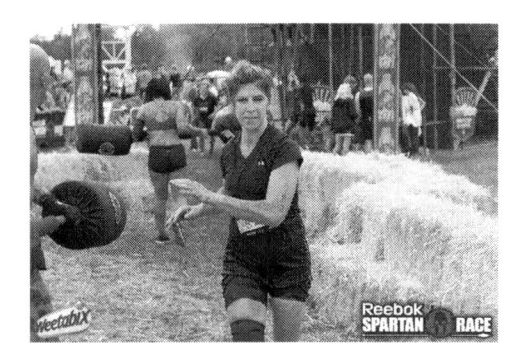

Dirty, sweaty, and unstoppable - embracing the challenges, one obstacle at a time at the Spartan Race. Fun times. Not fast times, fun times.

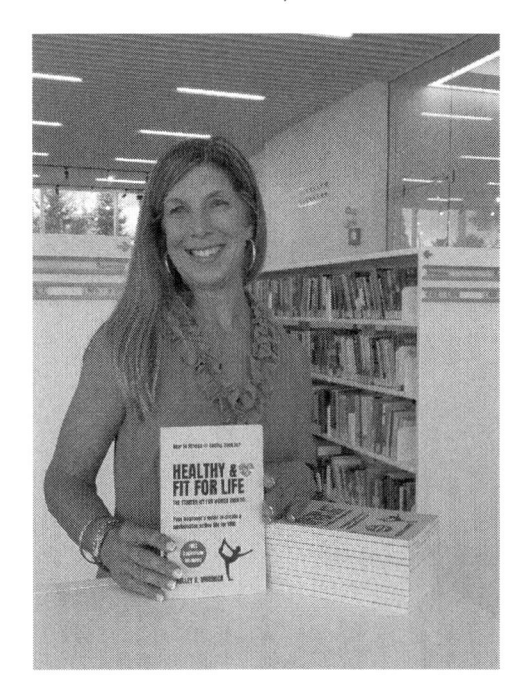

I'm a published author! Celebrating the launch of Book #1 - Healthy and Fit for Life.

> "Vulnerability is the birthplace of innovation, creativity, and change."
>
> - Brené Brown

CHAPTER 8
LET'S GET SOCIAL
– Cultivating Social Belonging

"Social inclusion and friendships – keystones of community – are what keep us active in the long run, promoting greater longevity and health."
– ParticipACTION

Humans are wired to connect. We benefit from being with others.

There is something truly special about connecting with others. Nurturing healthy and joyful relationships not only extends our lives but also enriches our well-being during those years.

One of my favorite places to experience this sense of community is Beyond Yoga Studio & Wellness Centre in Ottawa, Canada. As soon as you step through the door, the warm and inviting atmosphere surrounds you, filling the air with positive energy. People of all ages come together for tea, conversation, and camaraderie. The studio often buzzes with spontaneous knitting circles and lively discussions, where friends linger long after their classes have ended. The welcoming smiles and friendly greetings evoke the spirit of the beloved TV show "Cheers," but with a yogic twist. It's impossible to leave without feeling uplifted and inspired by the collective joy that fills the space.

Reflecting on the joyful people in my life, I see that they dedicate their time and energy to building community, both within their circles and beyond. These heart-centered, inclusive individuals prioritize engagement and connection, creating a positive impact that benefits us all.

When I think of people who cultivate happy relationships, two esteemed individuals come to mind: Roxanne and Yves. They have consistently dedicated their time to family, friends, and their community. Involvement has been a cornerstone of their lives, a value they instilled in their two daughters from an early age. Today, both daughters, now young women, are not only socially active but also professionally engaged in health and community care.

Full disclosure: Roxanne has been my dearest friend since we met in college in 1976. On our first day on campus, she took the initiative to introduce herself as we registered for classes, sparking a lifelong friendship that I cherish to this day.

Hopefully, we all have examples of heart-centered role models in our lives. If personal experiences don't illustrate the importance of social connections for our well-being, consider the insights of lifestyle medicine. This field of medicine teaches that strong social connections are essential for our health.

Good relationships can help prevent and treat chronic conditions such as obesity, diabetes, heart disease, cancer, and depression. Some psychologists even compare social connections to vitamins, suggesting we need "a dose of the human moment" just like we need vitamin C and D.

A study published by the *American Journal of Lifestyle Medicine* titled *The Connection Prescription* emphasizes the power of social interactions for health and wellness. The authors propose the idea of a "Connection Is Medicine" campaign, similar to the existing "Exercise Is Medicine" initiative, to highlight the value of social connections.

> *"'Incorporating social support and connections is critical for overall health and for healthy habits to be sustainable.'"*
>
> From a study published by the *American Journal of Lifestyle Medicine The Connection Prescription: Using the Power of Social Interactions and the Deep Desire for Connectedness to Empower Health and Wellness*
>
> Authors: Jessica Martino, Jennifer Pegg, Elizabeth Pegg Frates

Dr. Edward Hallowell, in his 1999 book Connect, underscored the importance of connections in our lives, describing them as a catalyst to feel part of something bigger, close to others, and welcomed and understood. He noted that even a brief five-minute conversation can significantly impact our well-being, provided both participants are fully engaged. Setting aside distractions and focusing on the person you're speaking with often leads to a positive response.

Our Prescription for Health

Consider that a five-minute conversation could serve as a prescription for health and longevity. In other words a Rx = Friendship. While building and maintaining friendships requires effort, the benefits make the extra work worthwhile.

LONGEVITY TAKEAWAYS

- ✓ Nurturing a Healthy Social Life: Longevity can greatly be enhanced by cultivating a healthy social life.

- ✓ Research-Backed Benefits: Strong social connections and supportive relationships contribute to better mental and physical health, lower stress levels, and a reduced risk of chronic diseases.

- ✓ **Community Engagement:** Engaging in social activities and feeling connected to a community boosts overall well-being and can help you live a longer, healthier life.

LONGEVITY CALLS TO ACTION

Here are some simple ways to weave more social interactions into your busy schedule:

1. **Schedule Social Time:** Just like you block off time for work or exercise, carve out specific times each week for socializing.

2. **Combine Activities:** Mix socializing with other activities—exercise with a friend, join a club, or attend local events together.

3. **Leverage Technology:** Keep in touch with loved ones through video calls, social media, or messaging apps. It's a great way to feel connected, no matter the distance.

4. **Attend Networking Events:** Get involved in professional gatherings or meetups to meet like-minded people and expand your social circle.

5. **Volunteer:** Find a cause you're passionate about. Volunteering is a fantastic way to meet new people and form meaningful connections.

6. **Join Groups:** Look for clubs or organizations that align with your interests or hobbies. It's a great way to bond over shared passions.

7. **Make Small Efforts:** Take advantage of little moments—chat with colleagues during breaks or strike up conversations with your neighbors.

8. **Prioritize Relationships:** Don't hesitate to reach out to friends and family regularly, even if it's just a quick text or phone call.

9. **Host Gatherings:** Invite friends over for casual get-togethers like dinner parties or game nights. It's a fun way to strengthen bonds.

10. **Balance Work and Social Life:** Set boundaries to ensure work doesn't overshadow personal time. Make it a priority to include social interactions in your routine.

By incorporating these strategies into your life, you can build meaningful relationships that enhance your well-being and longevity.

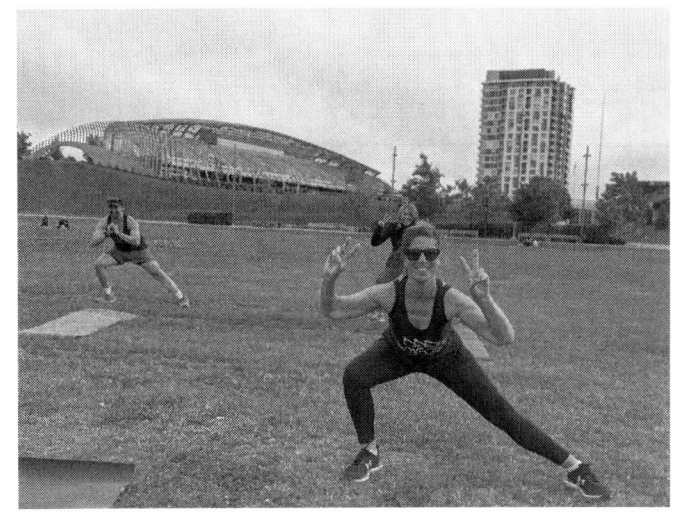

Moving with community at Movecamp Canada.

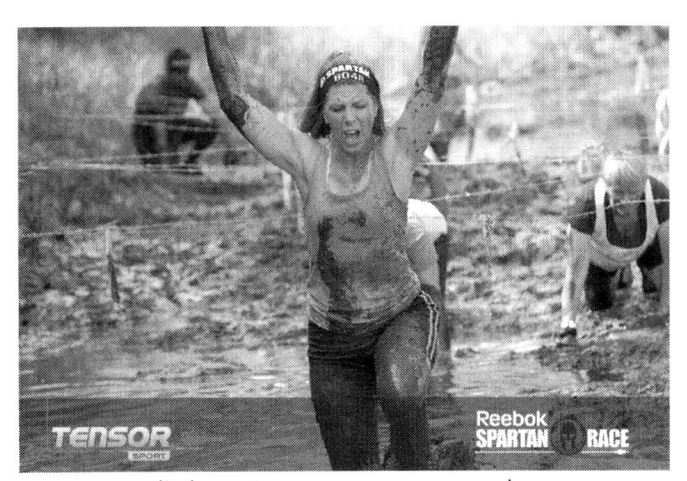

Just a little DIY spa treatment - mud, sweat, and a few tears of joy at a Spartan Race.

"The people you surround yourself with influence your behaviors, so choose friends who have healthy habits."

- Dan Buettner

CHAPTER 9
ALONE ZONE – SOLITUDE
The Real Self-Care Where Mindset Matters

"A calm mind brings inner strength and self confidence, so that's very important for good health."
– Dalai Lama

Solitude may be defined as a healthy, personal discipline that allows you to engage in meaningful self-reflection.

Taking some time for solitude is incredibly beneficial for your mental health. It gives you the opportunity to discover who you truly are, free from the influence of others. Embracing solitude allows you to reconnect with your authentic self.

Humans are social creatures, and we enjoy the company of others. We enjoy and benefit from the interactions with other people, emotionally and physically. This also brings some levels of stress, and often, we adjust our behavior based on the people around us, creating different versions of ourselves. This can be exhausting and emotionally draining if doses of quiet self-care moments are not injected.

Our hectic lives and hyper-distracted culture make it difficult to prioritize our emotional needs. Constantly glued to our screens for work and leisure, we have little time for boredom and creativity. However, the opportunity to be bored—having some free time when we're not busy or distracted—can actually be beneficial. When we allow ourselves to feel bored, we give our minds a chance to wander and think. This can lead to new ideas, problem-solving, and a deeper understanding of ourselves. In a world filled with constant activity and screen time, embracing boredom can help us become more creative and mindful.

As a child, I had the luxury of time to simply gaze at the clouds and indulge in daydreams. Those moments were incredibly relaxing, allowing me to appreciate my own company—an invaluable lesson my mother instilled in me. This skill has since been passed down to my children, and now it enriches the lives of our grandchildren as well. We are all avid readers and enjoy quiet reading time, which is something we do alone and sometimes together with our individual book. By exploring thought-provoking books and new topics that are challenging or inspiring, we give ourselves the gift of personal growth.

Enjoying your own company, or what my family refers to as our "Alone Zone," gives a sense of purpose and a time to reflect, which is beneficial for personal well-being and growth. To me, this is an opportunity to decompress, quiet my mind and rebalance. A daily practice of sitting with my own company, without the presence of others, even for a few minutes, has been beneficial for my emotional health and building my mental health resilience.

Building mental health resilience involves every aspect of our lives. It encompasses our thoughts and feelings, physical activity, nutrition, gut health, sleep, community connections, nature, spirituality, focus, and breathing. It is essential for each of us to prioritize self-care to nurture and sustain balance in body, mind, and soul.

Alone is not the same thing as loneliness. Loneliness is linked to negative health issues, isolation and depression. Loneliness is a health risk factor. Quality alone time feels like freedom and inspiration. To me it feels like ease and capacity has been created in my body and mind, where I can just be comfortable in my skin without any social pressures or obligations.

Finding peace and comfort in your own company is significant. Enjoying your time alone is a gift to yourself, and this is valuable to your mental health, your emotional needs, and your relationships with others. Are you comfortable doing things or just sitting in your own body without reaching out to someone for company?

Learning to be alone takes time, so try not to rush the process; do not put any pressure on yourself. The actions you take do not necessarily need to be big; they can be simple like journaling, or meditation, or going somewhere new each week and exploring places by yourself. Where could you find some quality "me" time in your schedule? What would that look like? First start by finding time in your schedule to build a routine (specific times, and staying consistent is key), limit the distractions and create a quiet space (turn off your devices or use noise-cancelling headphones), and perhaps even create a ritual to make it meaningful such as having a cup of tea or your favourite beverage while you engage in your solitude practice.

Finding quiet in the solitude of your own body—your original home—or being alone in your actual home where you live, or sitting in a park, alongside the water, are activities that may offer an approach that is appropriate for you.

How to start a fulfilling solitude practice?

- ✓ Read books that challenge your perspective or are about self-growth.

- ✓ Creativity – painting, drawing, playing music, or singing are wonderful ways to express yourself.

- ✓ Spend time in nature – walking, hiking, or simply sitting and enjoying nature and yourself.

- ✓ Include breathing exercises – to reduce stress and connect to your body like in yoga or mindfulness breathing.

- ✓ Explore cooking, baking, and gardening - these are fulfilling activities that allow you to engage your senses deeply. These solitary activities can bring joy and a sense of accomplishment.

LONGEVITY TAKEAWAYS

Taking care of your mental health is just as important as looking after your physical health. In fact, the two are deeply connected. Your stress levels can affect many aspects of your well-being, including your immune system, inflammation, sleep quality, and overall health habits. All of these factors play a significant role in your mental, emotional, and spiritual health.

Remember, taking care of your mind and spirit goes hand in hand with protecting your body. They work together in harmony, and by nurturing one, you can positively influence the other.

Be flexible and understand that your alone zone time may be interrupted, and it may not be perfect each time, so being adaptable to finding peace in the chaos of everyday life can simply be a moment or two at the checkout line—that is okay—we are incorporating strategies to enhance our mental well-being and self-awareness.

LONGEVITY CALLS TO ACTION

Your Five Practical Strategies for Finding Solitude in a Busy Life

1. **Find Small Windows of Time**

   - Micro-moments: Look for brief periods throughout your day—such as during your commute, lunch breaks, or while waiting in line—where you can practice solitude.

   - Consider waking up a bit earlier or staying up later to enjoy quiet moments before the day begins or after it winds down.

2. **Incorporate Solitude into Daily Routines**

   - Use your travel time for mindfulness exercises, like deep breathing or listening to calming music or podcasts.

   - Run errands alone, using that time to reflect or enjoy your own company.

3. **Schedule Solitude Time**

   - Block time in your calendar: Treat solitude like any other important appointment by scheduling it into your calendar. It will grow on you after a few times!

   - Weekly solitude sessions: Dedicate a specific time each week for a longer solitude session, whether it's a nature walk or a quiet afternoon at home.

4. **Create a Personal Sanctuary**

   - Set up a corner in your home that is solely for solitude – maybe a comfy chair and a window to gaze out.

   - Use noise-canceling headphones which allow you to focus inward and avoid other distractions.

5. Engage in Quick Mindfulness Practices

- Breath awareness: Take a few deep breaths whenever you feel overwhelmed to center yourself.

- Mini Meditations: Practice short meditation techniques, even for just a few minutes, during breaks or at your desk. Eating mindfully and walking meditation practices allow you to reflect and stay present.

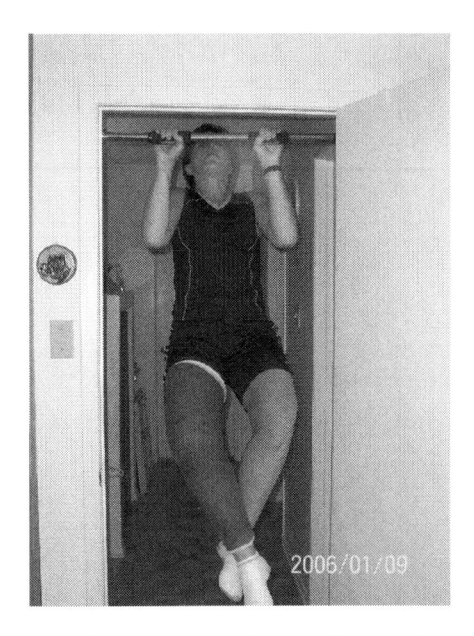

No excuses, just adaptations. Doing pull ups with a full leg cast.

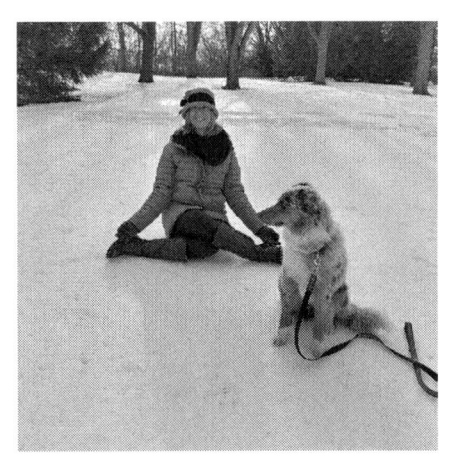

Snowga, fresh air and a loyal doggo - the perfect snow flow.

"Self-control is strength. Calmness is mastery. You have to get to a point where your mood doesn't shift based on the significant actions of someone else. Don't allow others to control the direction of your life. Don't allow your emotions to overpower your intelligence."

– Morgan Freeman

CHAPTER 10
EMBRACING HEALTHY DAILY HABITS FOR A HAPPIER LIFE

> "If you make your bed every morning, you will have accomplished the first task of the day. It will give you a small sense of pride and it will encourage you to do another task and another and another...Making your bed will also reinforce the fact that little things in life matter. If you can't do the little things right, you will never do the big things right...If you want to change the world, start off by making your bed."
> – Admiral William McRaven

Our habits and daily actions play a big part in shaping our lives. In the previous chapters, we have established that when we choose to develop good habits, we can improve our well-being, enhancing physical health, mental clarity, and emotional resilience. These practices provide us with a structure, a sense of purpose, and happiness.

I recently came across an insightful post on LinkedIn by a fitness trainer, Dan Go that resonated deeply with me. It highlighted some foundational habits that can significantly enhance our well-being:

> "Dear older generations,
>
> Waking up at 6 AM, tending to a garden, enjoying dinner at 5 PM, reading books, and going to bed at 9:30 PM feels amazing.
>
> I was wrong; you were right."

This perspective reminds us that sometimes the simple routines we once overlooked hold the key to greater energy and inner peace.

In gathering material for this book, I had the privilege of speaking with a diverse group of individuals from various ages and backgrounds. Their unique perspectives enriched our discussions on healthy habits and longevity, revealing how different experiences shape our approaches to well-being. Whether young professionals or retirees, each person contributed valuable insights, highlighting more commonalities than differences in their good habits.

A young entrepreneur named Tara, who is in her early 30s, shared her daily rituals and good habits. She begins each day with a little meditation, setting an intention and listing three things she's grateful for. After this mindful start, she emphasizes the importance of a healthy, protein-filled breakfast to fuel her day.

Tara looks forward to seeing her furry friends, no matter the weather. She believes that being outdoors not only clears the mind but also boosts her happiness levels. She said that as a child she was encouraged to discover at least one important lesson each day, a practice she maintains. She said that often it is the simplest of experiences that are a beautiful reminder to embrace each moment and approach life with curiosity!

This truly resonated with me. Eager to learn more, I decided to interview others to uncover their insights on the secret to longevity and the development of healthy habits.

One person I spoke with was an inspiring 84-year-old woman named Uschi (Ursula). I asked her to share her "secret sauce" for a happy, healthy life, and the secret behind her remarkable youthfulness and vitality.

Uschi emphasized that her daily habits and the principles instilled in her from a young age play a significant role in her well-being. She explained that she has consciously worked towards longevity throughout her life. Each day begins with a quiet meditation to set a positive tone, followed by a daily walk outdoors. Intrigued, I sought to learn more about how she and her 95-year-old husband, whom she has been married to for 64 years, maintain their happiness and mobility while living independently in a spacious home in the countryside—a lifestyle many of us aspire to at that age.

Uschi shared, "It starts at birth—the way we are raised, the genes we inherit, and the food we consume." While she acknowledged that genetics and luck play a part, she stressed the importance of the choices we make as adults. The food we eat, the exercise we engage in, and the responsibility we take for our health—such as regular doctor visits and appropriate medications—significantly impact our quality of life.

In her fifties, after her children had embarked on their own paths, Uschi developed an interest in holistic healing. She pursued courses and attended conferences to deepen her knowledge, ultimately becoming certified in holistic healing practices. This journey not only allowed her to help her community but also acquire a sense of accountability for her own health and well-being.

It's amazing how these small, everyday practices can lead to greater energy and peace of mind.

Jin-Jan (Janet) who is 89 years young, shared with me that her "secret sauce" to longevity lies in her deep connection to nature and her commitment to movement, particularly through yoga and gardening. As both an artist and a gardener, she finds joy in painting and nurturing flowers, whether in her garden or on canvas.

Having lived in her apartment for over 40 years, Jin-Jan dedicates her winter months to mending clothing for the elderly residents in her building. She also has a passion for fabric design, having studied at Cheltenham College of Art during her formative years from ages 14 to 16, a time she fondly recalls as some of the happiest of her life.

Despite her hands being gnarled and arthritic, her vibrant spirit and active mind drive her to help those in need. She is always smiling and radiates a delightful disposition.

In the summer, Jin-Jan keeps herself busy tending to 14 gardens, often with the assistance of one of her two daughters. Her love for gardening began at the age of eight while living in England, and she has since made it a point to create a garden wherever she has called home. "Wherever I have lived, I have created a garden," she remarked, reflecting her lifelong commitment to nurturing both plants and her community.

These three remarkable women, coming from different countries and varying in age, shared a set of similar habits that emerged as a common theme throughout my conversations with others.

What can we learn from their experiences? How can we cultivate more joy in our lives and start each day with a sense of calm and peace?

Here are some uplifting habits to consider as you create your own unique recipe for a fulfilling life:

1. **ESTABLISH A MORNING ROUTINE**

A consistent morning routine can brighten your entire day. Think of it like a menu: choose the elements that work best for you rather than trying to do everything. Here are some simple ideas to help you build a routine that fits your needs.

- **Wake Up at the Same Time:** Consistency helps regulate your body's internal clock, improving sleep quality and boosting energy levels.

- **Hydrate:** Start your day with a refreshing glass of water to rehydrate your body and kickstart your metabolism.

- **Practice Mindfulness or Meditation:** Spend a few minutes meditating or practicing deep breathing to calm your mind and prepare yourself for the day ahead.

- **Get Moving:** Engage in morning exercise—whether it's a workout, yoga, or a brisk walk. This movement releases endorphins that elevate your mood.

- **Enjoy a Nourishing Breakfast:** Fuel your body with a balanced meal rich in protein, healthy fats, and fiber to sustain your energy and sharpen your focus.

- **Engage Your Mind:** Set aside time for reading, journaling, or learning. This stimulates your brain and fosters a sense of accomplishment, especially in the morning.

- **Plan Your Day:** Review your to-do list and set intentions. Prioritizing tasks boosts productivity and provides clear direction.

- **Practice Gratitude:** Reflect on what you're thankful for, whether in a journal or through quiet contemplation. This simple act cultivates a positive mindset.

- **Prioritize Self-Care:** Take time for grooming or rituals that make you feel confident and ready to tackle the day.

- **Limit Distractions:** Avoid checking emails or scrolling through social media first thing in the morning. This helps you start your day with clarity and calmness.

Tips for Crafting Your Morning Routine

An effective morning routine equips you to feel energized and positive, setting the stage for a fulfilling day ahead. By embracing these habits, you'll cultivate a happier, more balanced life!

- **Start Small:** If you're new to routines, begin with one or two habits and gradually add more as you feel comfortable.

- **Personalize It:** Tailor your routine to fit your lifestyle and include activities that energize and inspire you.

- **Prepare the Night Before:** Lay out your clothes, plan your breakfast, and organize tasks to reduce morning stress.

- **Stay Flexible:** While consistency is important, allow yourself to adjust your routine as needed to keep it enjoyable and sustainable.

START SMALL - STAY CONSISTENT - ENJOY THE JOURNEY!

2. GRATITUDE PRACTICE

Taking a moment each day to reflect on what you're grateful for can boost your happiness and change your outlook.

See *CHAPTER 6: PRACTICE AND CULTIVATE GRATITUDE* for more details.

Here's how gratitude can transform your day:

- ✓ **Focus on the Positive:** Starting your day with gratitude helps you notice the good things in your life, lifting your mood and resilience.

- ✓ **Boost Mental Well-being:** Gratitude can lower stress and anxiety, promoting calmness and emotional stability.

- ✓ **Strengthen Relationships:** Appreciating others deepens connections and encourages kindness in your interactions.

- ✓ **Enhance Focus:** Recognizing what matters helps clarify your priorities, leading to better decisions and increased productivity.

- ✓ **Build Resilience:** Gratitude fosters a growth mindset, helping you see challenges as learning opportunities.

- ✓ **Support Physical Health:** Grateful people often adopt healthier habits, contributing to overall well-being.

Incorporating gratitude into your mornings cultivates a positive mindset, giving you enthusiasm and purpose throughout the day.

3. MINDFULNESS AND MEDITATION

In our fast-paced world, taking a moment to pause can do wonders for your stress levels and overall well-being. Incorporating mindfulness or meditation into your daily routine, even for just a few minutes, can bring about significant changes in your mental and physical health.

Top 3 Benefits of Mindfulness and Meditation

1. **Stress Reduction:**
   Mindfulness and meditation significantly lower stress levels by promoting relaxation and helping individuals manage anxiety, leading to a calmer mind and improved emotional well-being.

2. **Enhanced Focus and Clarity:**
   These practices improve concentration and mental clarity, allowing for better attention, increased productivity, and enhanced problem-solving abilities.

3. **Emotional Well-Being:**
   Mindfulness and meditation builds a greater sense of self-awareness and emotional regulation, promoting positive emotions, resilience, and a more balanced outlook on life.

I always incorporate meditation into my yoga classes because it nurtures compassionate, non-judgmental attitudes toward ourselves and others, which is fundamental to the practice of yoga. Another effective approach is to introduce a mantra into your daily routine. This simple practice can infuse your life with positivity, enhancing your sense of fulfillment and joy. After all, who wouldn't want more positivity in their life?

Here are three simple mantras for a healthy lifestyle:

1. *"I nourish my body and mind."*
   This mantra reinforces the importance of making healthy choices for both physical and mental well-being.

2. *"I embrace balance and moderation."*
   This encourages a balanced approach to eating, exercise, and self-care, promoting a sustainable lifestyle.

3. *"I am grateful for my health."*
   This mantra fosters a positive mindset and

appreciation for your body, helping to motivate healthy habits and self-care.

Metta Meditation: Loving Kindness Meditation (LKM)

"Metta is usually translated as 'loving kindness.' By practicing it you may find you are able to deal with situations with greater ease and lightness. I truly feel that it is a very empowering tool for transformations.

You can visualize, in the centre of your chest, your 'emotional heart,' an image of yourself as you are now or how you were as a child, perhaps supported by a loving mother. If visualizing is difficult, try just seeing your name written in the centre of your heart.

The metta practice starts with the pure intention that we wish to increase self-compassion from within. We may use the analogy of planting a seed, which we 'tend' through the practice until it grows into a beautiful flower or tree.

'May I be safe and protected.
May I be peaceful.
May I live at ease and with kindness'

In week two, after meditating on ourselves, we add somebody we love and care for:

'May you be safe and protected.
May you be peaceful.
May you live at ease and with kindness.'

Week by week we can expand the practice. We finally go still further, to include people we hardly know, or people who may have caused us irritation or hurt:

'May all beings be safe and protected.
May all beings be peaceful.
May all beings live at peace and with kindness.'

With this practice, we start with the mere intention of loving kindness, but experience has shown me that persisting with it can wonderfully enrich our lives. If every one of us just managed to touch one 'other' through this practice the world would indeed be a safer, kinder, and more peaceful place in which we live."

The Little Book of Mindfulness by Dr. Patrizia Collard

4. PHYSICAL ACTIVITY

Regular exercise is a cornerstone of a healthy lifestyle, boosting your mood and enhancing your overall well-being. Whether it's walking, yoga, or dancing, finding a form of movement you love can transform your life.

See *CHAPTER 4: AGING POWERFULLY STARTS NOW – Musclespan Matters* for more details.

Some key benefits of regular physical activity include but are not limited to :

- **Enhances Physical Health**

  - **Strengthens the Heart:** Regular exercise improves cardiovascular health, reducing the risk of heart disease and stroke.

  - **Maintains a Healthy Weight:** Daily physical activity helps manage weight, lowering the risk of obesity-related conditions.

  - **Builds Strength and Endurance:** Exercise increases muscle strength and endurance, making daily tasks easier and reducing injury risk.

  - **Boosts Immunity:** Regular movement enhances your immune system, helping you fend off illnesses.

- **Improves Mental Health**

  - **Lowers Stress and Anxiety:** Exercise releases endorphins, the body's natural stress relievers, helping to mitigate feelings of anxiety.

  - **Combating Depression:** Regular physical activity can be as effective as medication for managing mild to moderate depression.

For those with a family history of depression, exercise acts as a strong mood booster, helping to reduce symptoms and maintain emotional balance. Consistent workouts increase endorphins and provide a sense of accomplishment, making exercise an important tool for improving mental health and well-being.

- **Elevates Mood:** Exercise leads to both immediate and long-term mood improvements, keeping you energized and balanced.

- **Boosts Cognitive Function**

  - **Enhances Memory and Focus:** Regular physical exercise boosts cognitive function by increasing blood flow to the brain, enhancing memory, attention, and decision-making skills. It may also delay cognitive decline as we age, providing essential protection against dementia.

    As a caregiver to my mother, who suffered from Mixed Dementia and later Alzheimer's Disease, I witnessed the devastating effects of cognitive decline over twelve long years. This experience motivates me to promote fitness as a vital means of preserving brain health, so that others may avoid such a painful journey.

- **Promotes Better Sleep**

    - **Improves Sleep Quality:** Regular exercise helps you fall asleep faster and improves sleep depth, regulating your sleep-wake cycle and reducing insomnia symptoms for a more restorative rest.

    - **Alleviates Daytime Fatigue:** Improved sleep quality and increased energy from consistent exercise leads to greater wakefulness and alertness, keeping you energized and focused throughout the day—ready to tackle any challenges!

5. NOURISH YOUR BODY WITH BALANCED MEALS

A balanced diet rich in fruits, vegetables, and whole foods can positively impact your mood and energy levels. Implementing healthy daily eating habits can significantly improve your overall well-being and long-term health.

See *CHAPTER 5: NOURISH AND HYDRATE* for more details.

- ✓ Prioritize balanced meals
- ✓ Stay hydrated for optimal health
- ✓ Embrace mindful eating

Why It Matters:

Mindful eating helps you create a healthier relationship with food, helps reduce overeating, and increases your enjoyment of meals.

How to Practice Mindful Eating:

- **Savor Every Bite:**
  Take your time to chew and appreciate the flavors and textures of your food. This allows your body to recognize when it's full.

- **Eliminate Distractions:**
  Avoid screens while eating. Focus on your meal to enhance your dining experience. Concentrate on the flavours, textures, and aroma of the food, tune in, and fully enjoy your food.

- **Listen to Your Body:**
  Tune in to your hunger and fullness cues. Eat when you're genuinely hungry and stop when you feel satisfied.

6. CULTIVATE CONNECTIONS WITH LOVED ONES

Why It Matters: Building and maintaining strong relationships can significantly boost your happiness and longevity, enhancing your mental, emotional, and even physical health.

See *CHAPTER 8: LET'S GET SOCIAL – Cultivating Social Belonging* for details.

Benefits of Daily Relationship Practices:

- **Stress Relief:**
  Close relationships and connections provide emotional support, helping you manage life's challenges and reducing stress levels.

- **Mood Enhancement:**
  Regular interactions with loved ones can uplift your spirits and decrease the risk of depression.

- **Encouragement for Healthy Choices:**
  Friends and family can motivate you to adopt healthier habits, making it easier to stay on track with your health goals. Being accountable to someone helps you stick to your wellness goals. Find yourself a wellness pal!

- **Improved Physical Health:**
  Research shows that strong social ties can lead to lower blood pressure and a healthier heart.

- **Supportive Relationships:**
  Supportive relationships are crucial for living a long and healthy life. Studies have shown that having good friends and strong connections with others can significantly lower the chances of dying

early. In fact, lacking these healthy relationships can be just as harmful to your health as smoking or being overweight. This means that building and maintaining supportive relationships is essential for helping you live a longer life.

- **Sense of Purpose and Belonging:**
Strong relationships give your life meaning and purpose. Having people to care for and share experiences with creates a sense of belonging.

HOW TO BUILD STRONGER RELATIONSHIPS DAILY:

- ✓ **Reach Out:**
Make an effort to connect with friends or family each day, whether through a quick call, text, or visit.

- ✓ **Express Gratitude:**
Regularly acknowledge and appreciate the people in your life. This strengthens bonds and enhances emotional support.

- ✓ **Be Present:**
Engage fully in conversations, showing empathy and active listening.

- ✓ **Offer Support:**
Be there for loved ones when they need help or just someone to talk to, fostering deeper connections.

- ✓ **Share Activities:**
  Enjoy shared pastimes, whether it's cooking, walking, or playing games, to create lasting memories.

By prioritizing and nurturing your relationships daily, you create a strong social support system that will contribute to your health and a happier life. Remember to start small, stay consistent, and watch as these positive changes ripple through your well-being and your impact upon those that you love. A double whammy!

7. EMBRACE LIFELONG LEARNING: CULTIVATING HEALTHY HABITS FOR A CURIOUS MIND

Engaging in reading and learning not only stimulates your mind but also builds a sense of accomplishment and personal growth. By integrating these practices into your daily routine, you can enhance your knowledge, creativity, and overall well-being. Here are three effective strategies to make reading and learning a consistent part of your life:

Set Aside Dedicated Time

Why It Matters: Setting a regular time for reading and learning helps create a routine that seamlessly fits into your day; be flexible but do not skip it.

HOW TO DO IT

- **Morning Ritual:** Kickstart your day with 15-30 minutes of reading or learning. This could be during breakfast or your morning commute, setting a positive tone for the day ahead.

- **Evening Wind-Down:** Use reading as a calming activity before bed. This not only helps you relax but also reduces screen time, promoting better sleep.

- **Use Your Breaks:** Transform your work breaks or lunch hour into learning moments. Read an article, listen to an educational podcast, or watch a short, informative video.

Set Specific Learning Goals

Why It Matters: Clear goals keep you motivated and focused, making it easier to incorporate learning into your daily routine.

HOW TO DO IT:

- **Daily Reading Targets:** Challenge yourself to read a specific number of pages or chapters each day. For instance, aim for 20 pages each night.

- **Topic Exploration:** Select a subject or skill you're interested in and dedicate time each day to explore it further. This could involve reading books, taking online courses, or watching tutorials.

- **Track Your Progress:** Keep a journal or use an app to monitor your reading and learning achievements. This accountability can boost your motivation and highlight your growth over time.

Incorporate Learning into Daily Activities

Why It Matters: By weaving learning into your existing routines, you maximize your time and make continuous learning enjoyable.

HOW TO DO IT

- **Audiobooks and Podcasts:** Turn everyday tasks—like commuting or exercising—into educational experiences by listening to audiobooks or insightful podcasts.

- **Read in Small Increments:** Always have a book or e-reader handy. Use small snippets of time throughout the day—such as waiting in line or during short breaks—to read a few pages.

- **Join a Learning Community:** Get involved in online forums, book clubs, or study groups. Sharing what you learn with others not only reinforces your knowledge but also keeps you inspired.

Tips for Success

- **Choose Engaging Material:** Select books, articles, or courses that genuinely interest you. Enjoyment is key to sustainability.

- **Mix It Up:** Vary your learning methods by alternating between fiction and non-fiction, or balancing reading with videos and podcasts. Keeping it diverse keeps your curiosity alive.

- **Reflect on Your Learning:** Spend a few moments after each session to reflect on what you've read or learned. This helps reinforce the material and encourages you to apply it in your life.

By adopting these strategies, you can effortlessly integrate reading and learning into your daily life, paving the way for continuous personal and intellectual growth. Embrace the journey of lifelong learning and watch as it enriches your life in countless ways!

8. EVENING REFLECTION: A PEACEFUL END TO YOUR DAY

At the end of each day, taking a moment to reflect can be truly uplifting. Acknowledge your wins and pinpoint areas for growth to nurture a positive mindset. A calming evening routine not only helps you relax but also sets the stage for a great night's sleep. Here are three key elements to consider:

Reflection and Gratitude

- **Review Your Day:**
  Spend a few minutes thinking about what went well and what you can improve. This helps you process your day and let go of stress.

- **Practice Gratitude:**
  Before bed, jot down a few things you're thankful for. This simple act shifts your focus to the positive, boosting your mood.

Relaxation and Mindfulness

- **Engage in a Relaxing Activity:**
  Enjoy activities that help you unwind, like reading, taking a warm bath, or listening to soothing music.

- **Mindfulness or Meditation:**
  Spend a few minutes on mindfulness or meditation to calm your mind and reduce anxiety. Even simple breathing exercises can be effective.

Sleep Preparation

- **Consistent Sleep Routine:**
  Try to go to bed at the same time each night. This helps regulate your body clock for better sleep.

- **Create a Sleep-Friendly Environment:**
  Dim the lights and turn off screens at least 30 minutes before bed. Make your room cool and comfortable and consider calming rituals like sipping herbal tea. See the following section for more information.

Tips for a Smooth Evening Routine

- **Start Small:**
  Begin with one or two habits and gradually build from there.

- **Personalize Your Routine:**
  Choose activities that truly help you relax and reflect.

- **Be Consistent:**
  Stick to your routine regularly for the best results.

  By focusing on reflection, relaxation, and sleep preparation, you can end your day positively and set yourself up for tomorrow.

9. **SLEEP ROUTINE: PRIORITIZE RESTFUL SLEEP**

Getting quality sleep is essential for your overall well-being. To improve your sleep, try setting a consistent bedtime and creating a calming pre-sleep ritual. Incorporating some gentle exercises into your nightly routine can help you relax and increase flexibility, making it easier for your body to wind down for a restful night. Make sleep a priority, and you'll wake up feeling refreshed!

Relaxation Techniques Before Bed

Why: Engaging in relaxation techniques helps reduce stress and calm the mind, making it easier to transition into sleep.

HOW:

- ✓ Deep Breathing Practice - slows your heart rate and calms your mind.

✓ **Progressive Muscle Relaxation** - helps to release physical tension and promotes relaxation.

Include these relaxation techniques into your nightly routine to enhance your quality of sleep:

Gentle Stretching

WHY: Stretching before bed helps release tension in your muscles, improves flexibility, and promotes relaxation, making it easier to fall asleep.

HOW:

- **Forward Fold:**
  Stand with your feet hip-width apart, and slowly bend forward at the hips, reaching toward your toes. Let your head and arms hang heavy. Hold for 30 seconds to a minute, breathing deeply.

- **Child's Pose:**
  Kneel on the floor with your big toes touching and knees apart. Sit back on your heels, stretch your arms forward, and lower your forehead to the ground. Hold this position for a minute or longer, focusing on deep breathing.

- **Seated Spinal Twist:**
  Sit on the floor with your legs extended. Cross one leg over the other, placing the foot on the

outside of the opposite knee. Twist your torso toward the bent knee, using your opposite arm to gently deepen the stretch. Hold for 30 seconds on each side.

Deep Breathing (or Pranayama in yoga)

WHY:

Deep breathing exercises calm the nervous system, reduce stress, and signal to your body that it is time to relax and unwind.

HOW:

- **4-7-8 Breathing:** Sit or lie down in a comfortable position. Inhale quietly through your nose for 4 seconds, hold the breath for 7 seconds, and exhale completely through your mouth for 8 seconds. Repeat this cycle 4-8 times.

Legs Up the Wall (Viparita Karani Pose)

WHY:

This restorative yoga pose helps reduce swelling in the legs, relieves tension in the lower back, and promotes circulation, all of which can help you relax before bed.

HOW:

- Find a clear wall space and sit with one side of your body against the wall.

- Slowly lie back as you swing your legs up the wall, keeping them straight and close together.

- Your arms can rest at your sides, palms facing up, or on your abdomen.

- Hold this position for 5-15 minutes, focusing on deep, steady breaths.

Tips for Incorporating These Exercises

- **Set Aside Time:**
  Dedicate 10-20 minutes each night for these exercises. Doing them at the same time each evening can help establish a consistent routine.

- **Listen to Your Body:**
  Go gently with these exercises, especially if you are tired or new to them. The goal is to relax and unwind, not to push yourself too hard.

- **Combine with Your Evening Routine:**
  Pair these exercises with other evening habits, like brushing your teeth or reading, to create a seamless wind-down routine.

- **Avoid Stimulants:**
Limit caffeine, nicotine, and heavy meals before bed, as they can interfere with your ability to fall asleep.

- **Reduce Noise:**
Use earplugs, a white noise machine, or a fan to block out disruptive noises. A quiet environment promotes uninterrupted sleep.

These practical exercises can enhance your nightly routine by reducing physical tension, calming your mind, and preparing your body for a peaceful night's sleep.

However, falling asleep and staying asleep can be tough for many people, and several factors contribute to this struggle. Stress and anxiety, often fueled by worries about work or personal life, can lead to racing thoughts that keep us awake. Many of us have experienced the relentless grip of ruminating on a seemingly insignificant thought that can linger throughout the night, wreaking havoc on the following day.

A poor sleep environment—like exposure to artificial light from screens and disruptive noise—can also make it hard to get a good night's rest. Irregular sleep schedules, such as inconsistent bedtimes or shift work, can throw off our body's natural rhythms. Even lifestyle choices, like consuming caffeine or heavy meals before bed, along with health issues like insomnia and sleep apnea, can further complicate things.

The hormonal changes during menopause and pregnancy can lead to sleep disturbances. Additionally, as we age, our sleep patterns naturally change, often causing lighter sleep and more frequent awakenings.

By understanding these common challenges and addressing them, we can explore ways to improve our sleep quality and overall well-being.

It is important to seek medical advice if sleep difficulties persist, consult a healthcare provider to rule out or manage any underlying health conditions.

10. ACTS OF KINDNESS

> *"I've learned that people will forget what you said, people will forget what you did, but people will never forget how you made them feel."*
> *– Maya Angelou*

Small acts of kindness, whether for others or yourself, can boost your happiness and create a ripple effect of positivity. Integrating some of these habits into your daily life can gradually lead to increased happiness and a greater sense of fulfillment.

Kindness is a universal language that connects people and creates a sense of belonging. It feels good to be kind—it makes us feel connected and happy, creating a win-win situation.

Research shows that kindness boosts feel-good hormones like serotonin and dopamine, which can even lower blood pressure and stress. Best of all, kindness doesn't have to cost anything!

Top 10 Daily Kindness Habits

Here are ten simple ways to spread kindness each day:

1. **Give a Genuine Compliment:**
   A sincere compliment can boost someone's confidence and brighten their day.

2. **Help with a Task:**
   Offer a hand with small tasks like holding a door or carrying groceries to make someone's day easier.

3. **Send a Thoughtful Message:**
   Reach out to someone with a kind text or email to show you care.

4. **Listen Actively:**
   Give your full attention when someone speaks, showing you value their thoughts.

5. **Practice Gratitude:**
   Express thanks to those around you; it fosters positivity and strengthens bonds.

6. **Buy Someone a Treat:**
   Surprise someone with a small treat, like coffee or their favorite snack.

7. **Leave a Positive Note:**
   Write a kind note for someone to find, offering encouragement or a cheerful message.

8. **Donate Unused Items**
   Declutter and donate items you no longer need to help those in need.

9. **Pick Up Litter:**
   Help your community by picking up trash when you see it.

10. **Smile and Make Eye Contact:**
    A simple smile and eye contact can make someone feel seen and appreciated.

Try adding these small acts into your routine—they can make a big difference!

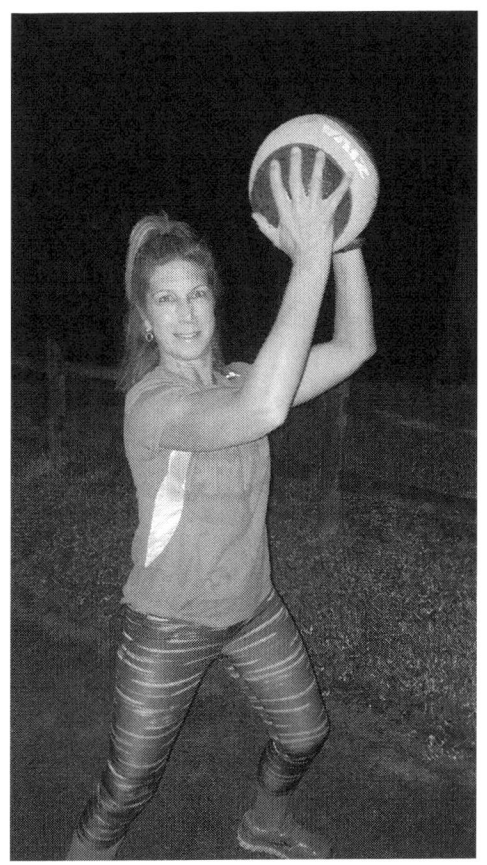

Medicine ball workout - throwing some weight around.

"Happiness is a Habit: Cultivate It."

- Ram Singhal

CHAPTER 11
MY 10 DAILY NON-NEGOTIABLES

"how to awaken your power

trust yourself
challenge your limiting beliefs
question your fears
ask yourself to grow

and remember that
you are the whole damn universe"

– spirit daughter

Daily habits can enhance your happiness and overall well-being. Positive habits can be cultivated and integrated into your life; all it takes is awareness and a commitment to practice them until they transform into consistent patterns. This process cannot be rushed, but it can be nurtured as you observe and perhaps marvel at the positive changes you feel.

It is important to recognize that developing good habits is a personal journey—what works for one person may not work for another, and progress can vary greatly; it is certainly not linear.

I live my life with three guiding principles: discipline, structure, and motivation. While I strive to maintain these habits for my well-being, I also embrace flexibility. Life occasionally leads us off course—whether it's staying up late or enjoying a glass of wine—but I believe in savoring those moments and then returning to my usual practices. It's all about finding balance: enjoying the present while staying committed to my health.

SHELL'S 10 HAPPINESS HABITS & RITUALS

1. **Morning Rituals**

    Every morning, I embrace the day with a series of uplifting rituals that set a positive tone. Here's how I start:

    Stretching and Breathing Exercises: I begin with a few gentle stretches to wake up my body:

    - Floor Sweepers
    - Cat and Cows
    - Standing Arcs
    - Seated Straddle Side-to-Side Push-ups

Welcoming the Day: I open the curtains wide, letting in the morning light while verbally greeting the day. It's a simple but powerful way to embrace the new possibilities ahead.

Honoring Family: As I pass by the much-loved photo of my mom and mother-in-law, I take a moment to say "good morning" to them. It's a lovely way to feel connected to my roots.

Playtime with Bailey Boops: Our playful Australian Shepherd brings so much joy to my mornings. Her happy energy is contagious and always makes me laugh.

These might sound a bit quirky, but these small acts fill me with positivity and put a smile on my face before I even step into the kitchen.

2. **Daily nutrition practices**

- Breakfast 20-30 g protein, cup of hot tea/coffee
- Mid-morning – snack (fruit)
- Lunch – 20-30 g protein, raw vegetables
- Mid-afternoon – apple with natural peanut butter
- Supper – 30g protein, lots of greens and vegetables

I am committed to my food choices and genuinely enjoy what I eat. I take the time to savor each meal, appreciating the flavors, and I refuse to rush through the experience or eat something that does not fit my requirements. Nutrition is a priority for me. I make it a point to focus on my meals and ensure I'm nourishing my body in a way that feels right for me whether at home, in restaurants, or during a visit.

3. **Hydrate – "Be like water.", Bruce Lee**

   I make it a priority to stay hydrated throughout the day. Each morning, I start by drinking 24 ounces (three cups) of water before having anything else. I continue to drink several glasses throughout the morning, afternoon, and evening. Since my job is quite physical and I often teach hot yoga, I find myself drinking even more water as the day goes on. Staying hydrated is essential for me!

4. **MOVE: Get Physical and Keep Moving**

   Every day is filled with movement—whether it is a workout, resistance training, range of motion exercises, or a yoga practice. I focus on pushing, pulling, and lifting during these sessions, which are dedicated to my own fitness, not just my students or clients.

As a fitness instructor and personal trainer, I may teach and demonstrate movements anywhere from three to five classes each day and have a few clients depending on my schedule. To prepare, I practice each routine the day before and again on the day of the class. This helps keep the workouts fresh in my mind so I can effectively support my students—it's their workout, after all—but I also get in an extra workout for myself in the process. This is my bonus!

- I average 10-14k steps a day, walking the dog and taking daily walks wearing my weighted vest. Some days it is 9k and others it is 18k; I take into consideration my class load and fatigue level and do not get hung up on the number of steps.

- Dead arm hang is a daily practice for me. It is a simple yet effective exercise that boosts shoulder mobility, grip strength, and helps relieve back pain. They engage key muscles, improve posture, and decompress the spine, making them beneficial for everyone. I find it especially restoring after a long teaching day; it helps decompress my muscles and leaves me feeling significantly better overall.

I encourage all my classes to try the dead arm hang to experience its benefits for back health and overall wellness. This exercise can be easily modified to suit different fitness levels—for instance, beginners can start with shorter hangs or perform the exercise with bent knees and feet on the ground as they build strength.

From one of my social media posts, "Trust me, you want to be THE big pickle jar opener in your family. Grip strength IS longevity."

So why does Shell keep posting about doing a daily 2-minute Dead Hang?

SHORT STORY

- Grip strength
- Decompresses the spine
- Shoulder mobility
- Stretches the upper body

HOW TO DO IT

A dead arm hang is a simple yet effective exercise that helps improve grip strength and shoulder stability. Here's how to do it:

1. **Find a Bar:** Locate a sturdy pull-up bar or any overhead bar that can support your weight. *The playground structure is ideal as you take your daily walks.

2. **Grip the Bar:** Stand under the bar and reach up to grab it with both hands, using an overhand grip (palms facing away) or an underhand grip (palms facing you). Your hands should be shoulder-width apart.

3. **Hang:** Jump or step off the ground to let your body hang freely from the bar. You can also use a riser in the gym. Keep your arms straight and engage your shoulders slightly to avoid excessive strain.

4. **Position Your Body:** Let your legs hang straight down, keeping your body relaxed. Avoid swinging; stay as still as possible.

5. **Hold:** Maintain this position for as long as comfortable, aiming for 20-60 seconds. Focus on your breathing and try to relax your upper body.

6. **Release:** When you're finished, carefully step or jump back to the ground to release your grip.

Tip: Start with shorter hangs and gradually increase the duration as your grip strength improves. If you are in the gym, always ensure your safety by using a mat or having a spotter if you're unsure.

LONG STORY

Dead hang is a forearm and grip strength exercise, and practice. It will help the ability to hold your body weight; the longer you can hold on, the stronger your grip becomes. There are over 20 muscles in your forearms FYI.

Many of the activities and movements that occur in our lifestyles often compress our spine; think of sitting in front of the computer. Even our workout exercises and activities such as lifting heavy objects and squatting compress the spine.

Dead hangs can decompress the spine as gravity pulls you down, and hanging helps to lengthen and decompress your spine. Your body's weight gently pulls your vertebrae apart, enabling your discs to expand, which can help relieve any back pain or tension you may have.

This will give your shoulders, arms, and back muscles a nice stretch. It will improve your shoulder health by increasing its range of motion. A great stretch for your latissimus dorsi muscles/ your lats ….think bodybuilders and the big back muscles that "accordion" out when they pose.

So come hang with me. Try 15-second increments. Work your way up. Simple.

5. **ALONE ZONE TIME: Prioritize time to be with yourself**

   - Morning Meditation: I begin my day by dedicating a few moments to sit quietly, breathe deeply, and clear my mind through meditation. Even a brief session of a few minutes can be incredibly beneficial, bringing a sense of peace and clarity.

   - Gratitude Practice: I take time to express gratitude for the people and things in my life, helping to set a positive tone for the day. For me this does not need to be an extensive list; sometimes, I focus on just one person or experience, reflecting on its significance and impact.

   - Every day I love to spend some quiet time to read a book (one I can hold in my hands), even a few pages shift my thoughts and mood for the better.

   - I set aside time each day to watch the birds at my feeders. It's a wonderful mix of entertainment and peace, creating a calming and soothing experience. I enjoyed this activity as a child, and it has become a cherished daily ritual.

Interestingly, when I struggled with depression years ago, my therapist suggested that I take a moment to pause, observe the birds, breathe deeply, and focus on the present moment. This is the time to just be with myself and clear out the cobwebs of the day.

6. **BE WITH THE PEOPLE YOU LOVE – Get social and enrich your life**

   Spending time with family and friends is essential for me. Having people I can rely on—and who can rely on me—plays a vital role in our human experience, creating a sense of connection and purpose.

   I am lucky that my kid-adults and grandkids live in the area, so we visit often. However, each morning, we reach out to each other on our family chat just to say HI and check in. Everyone has busy lives - how lucky are we that there is technology for facetime! This is a morning ritual that is deeply appreciated. Driveway quick visits or tuck n' roll hugs are sometimes our only option, but we all make it work.

   As a fitness instructor, my job is incredibly social, and I feel fortunate to spend so much time surrounded by happy, like-minded individuals.

The energy we create together is truly amazing! I really love the opportunities to connect with friends, colleagues, and clients, sharing the ups and downs of life–the good, the bad and the ugly. And whether we're laughing, celebrating joyful moments, or experiencing deeper emotions, these experiences make my journey even more rewarding.

7. **Find Your Purpose**

   Each day brings me an opportunity to do something purposeful. I am driven by goals and checklists as it makes me feel useful.

   - What is my ONE purpose or goal for the day? What do I want to achieve?
   - How does it align with my life goals? Or does it?

8. **Gratitude and Give Back to My Community**

   Every day, I embrace gratitude through my yoga practice and teaching.

   I see each day as a chance to spread positivity—whether it is through a smile, a compliment, or a willingness to lend a hand. Volunteering doesn't always have to be formal; there are countless opportunities around us. Sometimes, it is as simple as dedicating time to a student after class, sharing insights on wellness and fitness.

I am fortunate to have a wonderful circle of friends. We uplift each other by sharing our diverse services across our networks, whether through social media or newsletters. We are each other's cheerleaders, always showing up to support one another.

I really enjoyed the book, Be Useful: Seven Tools for Life by Arnold Schwarzenegger, the world's greatest bodybuilder, in which he shares his tool kit of seven rules to realize your true purpose in life. The book offers practical advice on goal setting, risk-taking, and making a positive impact. Arnold highlights the importance of serving others—BE USEFUL. I take that thought to heart.

9. Evening Routine & Mindfulness

My recipe is pretty simple and takes very little time to set the stage for a good night's sleep.

- Gratitude practice – 2 minutes
- Stretching and breath practice – 2 minutes
- Meditation practice – 2 minutes
- Read a few pages of a book to change the narrative of a busy mind.

10. Rest and Sleep Routine

- I try to go to bed at the same time each night – the key word is try.
- I wake up at the same time each morning.
- I give myself permission to rest, let go of the day, so that I can rest my body, brain, and emotions and replenish fully.
- I know that rest is the most important thing we can do for ourselves, and that we undervalue its importance and we overvalue "doing." I continue to work on this but I struggle like many of us.

For me it is ultimately about balance, savoring the present while remaining committed to my health and well-being.

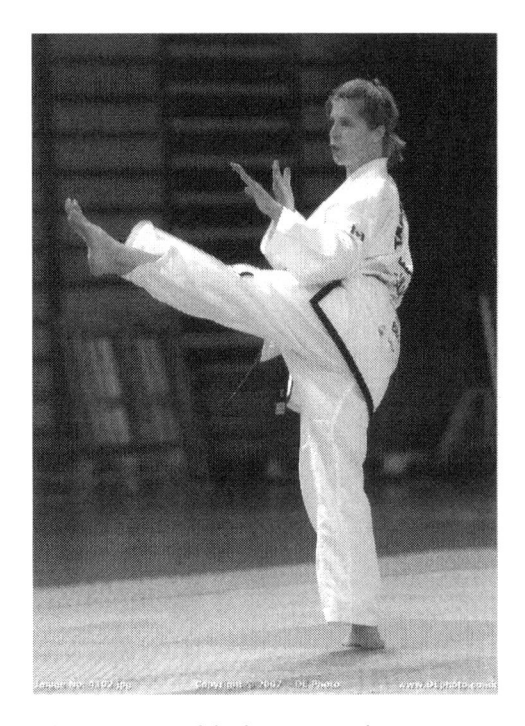

ITF Taekwondo 2007 World Championships at 47 years young.

"I have learned that as long as I hold fast to my beliefs and values - and follow my own moral compass - then the only expectations I need to live up to are my own."

- **Michelle Obama**

CHAPTER 12
AUTHOR'S NOTES AND LONGEVITY HACKS N' TIPS

"Living longer and feeling better is the sum of a few small easy choices you can incorporate into everyday life."
– Dan Buettner

We cannot force change. When we want to change, we will change.

Cultivating a nurturing environment for positive habits is not a linear journey, and it can be challenging and frustrating too. Developing new, positive, and healthier habits requires time and energy. Breaking away from unhealthy patterns can be even more challenging than building them.

As humans, we often fall into the trap of self-judgment and harsh criticism. When I catch myself slipping into self-criticism, I take a moment to pause and remind myself to speak kindly to myself, just as I would to 4-year-old me. I find that this gentle self-talk can transform my mindset. When going through a rough patch recently, I replaced my phone screen saver with a photo of a 4-year-old me. That was highly effective and reminded me to move forward without any guilty feelings.

Take a moment to reflect on your thoughts and choose kindness and self compassion vs. negative self-talk. There is a reason for the wonderful mantra, "Always choose kindness." Choosing kindness has a positive impact on both you and those around you.

Our intention of creating healthier habits is to find personal joy and well-being in life now and for the future. Empowering us to grow as a whole person - body, mind, and soul.

> **MINDSET CHECK AND MANTRA**
>
> *"I prioritize progress over perfection and have let go of the all-or-nothing mentality. This mindset shift is crucial to my long-term success."*

Here are five easy tips you can add to make your longevity journey easier and smoother:

1. SOCIAL TIP: FIND YOUR TEAM & SURROUND YOURSELF WITH LIKEMINDED PEOPLE

Volunteer in your community and offer your services to make life better for others. In turn your life will vastly improve, and you will feel happier. The collective is always a great place to be! As Arnold Schwarzenegger says, "Be useful."

When I felt there was a need for social connection, I found outdoor fitness groups that offered free fitness. Each time I showed up, I was greeted and welcomed. It became a great way to find like-minded people who enjoyed being outdoors all four seasons, who enjoyed working out in the snow and playing; it created a sense of belonging, and when you missed a week folks noticed. There was a feeling of "show up," an expectation from the group. In Ottawa we have a number of free fitness groups across the city, on different days of the week, which allows for multiple opportunities to find your people (often they overlap!). I decided to replicate the formula and create my own weekly free family-fitness workout and free yoga in the summer in my own community. It was so rewarding personally, and it gave me a sense of purpose to volunteer my passion, connect with neighbours in a meaningful way, and enjoy our beautiful park which was underused except for hockey in the winter.

Who inspires you to be your higher self to build and maintain habits to keep you on track with your longevity habits and goals? Reach out to your friends and family to support you as you incorporate new habits and release ones that no longer serve you.

Joining a walking group is the easiest way to get moving and meet people. If you do not have one in your community then start one.

COMMUNITY = as I the individual am the lower-case i. We are all in this together. Your healthy habits will influence your social circle to improve theirs too.

I want to give a huge shoutout to MOVE CAMP Canada (MC) and my amazing fellow MC coaches. They've become some of the sweetest friends I could ever ask for—always there with a smile and ready to support me in all my fitness endeavors. We genuinely share our skills and expertise to uplift each other and our clients. I mean, who else would throw me a 65th birthday party with planks as the main party game? That's the kind of camaraderie we have!

2. NUTRITION TIPS & HACKS: MAKE FOOD & NUTRITION SIMPLE

- ✓ Whether in-person or online, perhaps there are ways you can mitigate your way through nutrition obstacles by engaging a nutritionist or registered dietitian vs. reaching for takeaway.

For example, my friend Sarah Boyd, a dedicated Nutrition Coach and Personal Trainer, believes that navigating the world of nutrition doesn't have to be overwhelming. To help her clients discover the best ways to nourish their bodies, Sarah emphasizes four core principles for them to embrace:

1. **Variety in Foods:** Incorporate a diverse range of foods for optimal nutrition.

2. **Portion Control:** Be mindful of serving sizes to maintain balance.

3. **Balanced Bites:** Aim for a harmonious mix of macronutrients in every meal.

4. **Gradual Change:** Embrace small, incremental adjustments for lasting results.

You can follow Sarah on Instagram at @sarah_thehealthcoach.

- ✓ My friend Samantha Moonsammy-Gordon is an incredibly busy professional, balancing several senior roles as well as being an event speaker, publisher, and author, all while raising young children. Understanding the importance of nutrition for her family's well-being, she and her husband work together to prepare batches of healthy meals so they can have them for a few nights or for lunch too. They always keep plenty of freshly cut fruits and vegetables on hand, along with hummus and other nutritious dips.

- ✓ Samantha mentioned that there are times when the kids need to eat in the car on the way to after-school activities. To make this easier, they've created a go-tray with compartments that sit comfortably on the kids' laps, filled with their favorite healthy snacks and meal leftovers. This approach is a much better option than stopping at a fast food drive-thru. What an effective and efficient way to deliver good food to kids, and reduce a parent's stress level,

- ✓ Generally, as a society, we all eat far too much; it would be ideal to consider moderating our total food intake. By reducing the size of the dinner plate, we can adjust our quantity, and by focusing on our meals and enjoying time together, we eat slower and taste our food.

3. FITNESS TIPS: EMBRACE HOME WORKOUTS FOR A FLEXIBLE ROUTINE

Problem: Insufficient time to go to the gym? Consider the economics of a home workout might be your answer.

Consider: Time/Busy Schedule. What is your time worth?

- ✓ In today's fast-paced world, many people struggle to fit gym visits into their busy schedules. A home workout can be a practical and effective solution that allows you to stay fit without the hassle of commuting.

  With countless online fitness programs available for all fitness levels, you can easily find routines that suit your preferences and goals.

- ✓ Additionally, consider hiring a personal trainer who can come to your home. This option not only provides the expertise of a professional but also tailors workouts to your specific needs, ensuring you get the most out of your sessions.

  Many trainers also offer partner training, which allows you to share the experience with a friend, partner, or neighbor. This not only makes the workouts more enjoyable but also makes it more economical, as you can split the cost.

✓ When evaluating your fitness options, consider these key economic factors:

1. **Time Value:** How much is your time worth? Home workouts eliminate travel time, allowing you to maximize your schedule.

2. **Cost Efficiency:** Compare the costs of gym memberships, classes, and personal training. With home training, you may find more affordable options, especially when sharing sessions with a workout buddy.

3. **Convenience:** Working out at home means you can exercise whenever it fits your schedule, making it easier to stay consistent.

The story behind my in-home training business emerged from a real need I observed in many people's lives. After COVID-19, it became clear that a lot of individuals were struggling to maintain or even start a workout routine. With changing work schedules and the return to the office, the once easy opportunity to squeeze in a workout during the day disappeared.

Many found it challenging to commit to a gym visit, and the convenience of exercising at home during a break—without the need for daycare—was gone. As a result, some people who had never made it to the gym faced health issues, lost muscle and strength, and experienced significant weight gain.

Recognizing these challenges, I wanted to offer a solution that empowers everyone to get moving again, right from the comfort of their homes. My goal is to make fitness accessible and enjoyable, no matter your circumstances. "Let's work together to get you back on track!" is the plan I share with my clients.

By understanding these factors, you can make informed decisions about your fitness routine that align with your lifestyle and budget. Embrace the flexibility of home workouts and take charge of your fitness journey today!

4. FITNESS TIP: THE POWER OF A WORKOUT BUDDY

Having a workout buddy can significantly enhance your fitness journey, regardless of your age or fitness level. In my experience offering at-home training, I've found that partnering up makes workouts not only more enjoyable but also creates a sense of accountability.

When it comes to staying committed to your fitness routine, working out with a friend can make all the difference. Unlike going to a gym solo or following an online program, having a workout buddy creates a special bond that keeps you accountable. You're much more likely to show up and give it your all when someone else is relying on you!

So, why not find a workout partner and enjoy the motivation and fun that come from pursuing fitness goals together? A huge shout-out to my amazing training partners who have kept me on track: my running buddies Lynn and Fiona, my workout companion and fellow Spartan competitor Sheila, and the incredible women in the competitive Taekwon-Do team where we really left it all on the mat . And let's not forget my favorite free-fitness crew, The Arboretum Hill Club, who brave the elements every Friday at 6:29 AM for outdoor workouts. Together, we tackle hills and enjoy fun fitness sessions all year round!

5. STRESS REDUCING TIP: PUT AWAY TECHNOLOGY – Your Phone – and Reduce Stress

When you get home, try putting your phone away. Cutting down on phone use in the evening can help you enjoy more quality time with your family and reduce stress.

Remember, your time with loved ones is what matters most! Unless something urgent comes up, give yourself permission to "step away from the cell." Take this opportunity to relax, connect, and unwind without the distractions of notifications and social media. You'll feel much better for it!

6. FIND YOUR PURPOSE – Share Your Gift with the World - Your Community

We all know that having a sense of purpose or meaning in life is closely tied to longevity and happiness. This understanding can be a powerful motivator for us to contribute in meaningful ways. Think about how you can share your time and talents—whether through your work, volunteer efforts, or simply by being a supportive friend or family member. Discovering your purpose isn't just about personal fulfillment; it's about creating a life filled with authenticity and joy, where each day feels significant.

To give you some background, my mom was living with mixed dementia, and I spent over six hours a day caring for her. During this time, I was also leading a professional team, trying to be there for my husband and family, and fitting in my long-distance runs and workouts. Life can throw unexpected challenges our way; Alzheimer's disease is relentless, and I knew things would only get harder. Eventually, I reached a breaking point. My schedule felt overwhelming, and I realized I couldn't keep going like this—something had to change, and that something was me.

At 57, I made a significant decision to change careers. I went back to school to get all my certifications so I could follow my lifelong passion for teaching fitness and yoga. Since then, my purpose and joy have become clear. I chose to follow my heart, and that choice has made all the difference.

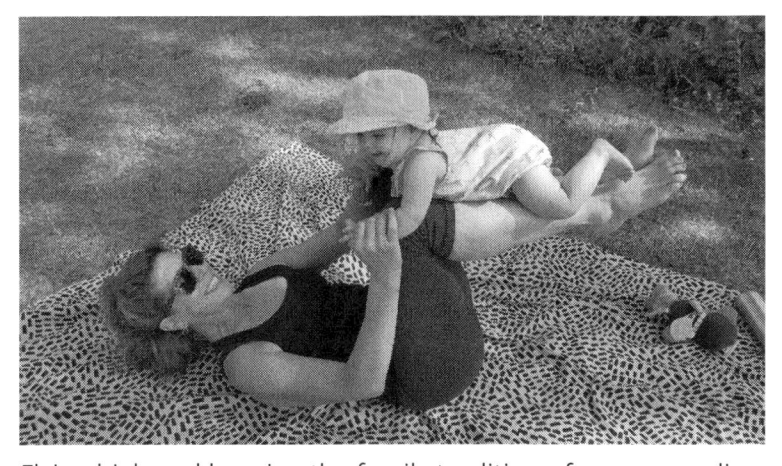

Flying high and keeping the family tradition of acro yoga alive. Granddaughter Shae and Nana.

"First, create little goals for yourself. Don't worry about the big, broad stuff for now. Focus on making improvements and banking achievements one day at a time."

- Arnold Schwarzenegger,
Be Useful: Seven Tools for Life

CHAPTER 13
EMBRACING LIFE WITH MY LIFE CALENDAR

I want to share something truly transformative that has touched my heart and reshaped my perspective: the Life Calendar. This powerful visual tool has become a beacon in my journey, helping me feel grounded, set meaningful goals, and honor my achievements.

Imagine, if you will, each box on the calendar representing a week of your life—a vivid reminder of the precious time we have, from the moment we take our first breath to the twilight years of our lives. As I dedicate just five quiet minutes to reflection, I trace each box, and in that simple act, I am reminded to cherish every fleeting moment with those I love.

This isn't just a practical exercise; it's a heartfelt wake-up call. It encourages me to embrace life fully and focus on what truly matters. The Life Calendar breaks down the complexities of our existence into a tangible format, allowing me to reflect deeply, prioritize with intention, and find clarity on the path I wish to walk.

At its core, this tool is a celebration of life—a gentle nudge to live fully and meaningfully. It invites us to pause, to breathe, and to really consider how we spend our time.

If you're seeking a way to deepen your connection with your own journey and to celebrate each step along the way, I wholeheartedly encourage you to embrace this practice.

Let it inspire you to reflect, to grow, and to truly savor the beautiful gift of life.

SHELLEY'S LIFE IN WEEKS

FOSTER GRATITUDE EVERY DAY

"Stop waiting for the right time.

Waiting to feel ready or a little less afraid.

Waiting for someone to come along and tell you that today is the day to start.

The problem with waiting is no one is coming.

The only permission you need is your own."

- Mel Robbins

CONCLUSION
Transform Your Life Today!

Are you ready to embark on a journey of self-discovery and lasting change?

In Search of Longevity is your guide to reshaping your life through the power of healthy habits. Imagine the profound impact of prioritizing exercise and mindfulness—not just on your physical health, but on your emotional resilience and overall happiness.

As you embrace this transformative path, you'll not only enhance your own well-being but also inspire those around you. Together, we can create a ripple effect of positivity and health in our communities.

Remember, sustainable health isn't just a dream; it's an achievable reality for everyone.

Let's take the first step together!

xxoo
Shell

RESOURCES

ARTICLES

- ✓ *Brainwork: The Power of Neuroplasticity*, for Health Essentials from Cleveland Clinic, psychologist Grace Tworek https://health.clevelandclinic.org/neuroplasticity

- ✓ Medical News Today - 5 neuroplasticity exercises to try https://www.medicalnewstoday.com/articles/neuroplasticity-exercises

- ✓ *Building Healthy Habits When You're Truly Exhausted* by Elizabeth Grace Saunders
  Harvard Business Review
  https://hbr.org/2022/04/building-healthy-habits-when-youre-truly-exhausted

- ✓ Implausibility of radical life extension in humans in the twenty-first century
  - Authors S. Jay Olshansky, Bradley J. Willcox, Lloyd Demetrius & Hiram Beltrán-Sánchez
  natural aging journal October 2024
  https://www.nature.com/articles/s43587-024-00702-3

BOOKS

- ✓ *OUTLIVE* – Dr. Peter Attia

- ✓ *Forever Strong – A New, Science-Based Strategy for Aging Well* – Dr. Gabrielle Lyon

- ✓ *Growing Young* – Marta Zaraska

- ✓ *Atomic Habits: An Easy & Proven Way to Build Good Habits & Break Bad Ones* - James Clear

DOCUMENTARY

- ✓ *Live to 100: Secrets of the Blue Zones* - documentary by Dan Buettner. The new doc series travels around the world to investigate the diet and lifestyles of those living the longest lives.

PODCASTS

- ✓ The Peter Attia Drive Podcast
  The Drive is hosted by Dr. Peter Attia, a Stanford/Johns Hopkins/NIH-trained physician focusing on the applied science of longevity, the extension of human life and well-being.
  https://www.youtube.com/playlist?list=PLIFIZLYiJ88Pnq_MSHfRH5KsX07XXTdL_

- ✓ Peter Attia MD Drive Podcast
  Exercise for aging people: where to begin, and how to minimize risk while maximizing potential
  https://www.youtube.com/watch?v=Yz0W-P0UaKE&t=51s

- ✓ We no longer know how to make humans live longer – only better
  CBS Radio Quirks & Quarks with Bob McDonald Episode November 29, 2024 - https://www.cbc.ca/radio/quirks/nov-30-exploring-the-limits-of-human-longevity-and-more-1.7395863

WEBSITES

- ✓ Oprah and Dr. Peter Attia Get Real About Living Better for Longer
  https://bit.ly/3NL4IzW

- ✓ Atomic Habits: How to Get 1% Better Every Day - James Clear
  https://www.youtube.com/watch?v=U_nzqnXWvSo&t=70s

- ✓ ParticipACTION

  - Aging
    https://www.participaction.com/the-science/explore-benefits/aging/

- Community
  https://www.participaction.com/the-science/explore-benefits/community/

✓ *Changing Your Habits for Better Health*
  National Institute of Diabetes and Digestive and Kidney Diseases
  https://www.niddk.nih.gov/health-information/diet-nutrition/changing-habits-better-health

✓ McMaster Optimal Aging Portal
  https://www.mcmasteroptimalaging.org/

VIDEOS

✓ Make Health Last - Canadian Heart & Stroke Foundation
  https://www.youtube.com/watch?v=qNkzVz5Aljk

✓ McMaster Optimal Aging Portal
  Exercise: Powerful Medicine for Health and Aging with kinesiology researcher Dr. Stuart Phillips
  https://www.mcmasteroptimalaging.org/blog/detail/videos/2023/01/25/exercise-powerful-medicine-for-health-and-aging

✓ Orthopedic Surgeon and Longevity Expert Dr. Vonda Wright talks about the Keys to Active Aging
  https://www.youtube.com/watch?v=ZK481WtfyL0

- ✓ Dr. William Li - YouTube Channel
  World-renowned physician, scientist, speaker, and NYT Bestselling author of "Eat To Beat Disease."
  https://www.youtube.com/@DrWilliamLi

- ✓ Dan Buettner: Live to 100 with secrets of the blue zones | Professor Tim Spector, Professor of Genetic Epidemiology
  https://www.youtube.com/watch?v=ImgSREOjFH4

- ✓ TEDx - Embrace Age with a Longevity Mindset | Helen Hirsh Spence
  https://www.youtube.com/watch?v=SwhOQRduE7c&t=1s

- ✓ TEDxBocaRaton - Your socks may hold the key to aging better | Carole Blueweiss
  https://www.youtube.com/watch?v=6F6m9CGFnk0

- ✓ How to make or break a habit with the 4 Laws of Behavior Change | Peter Attia, M.D. with James Clear
  https://www.youtube.com/watch?v=zCkHtvu8Fs4

MEET SHELLEY A. MURDOCK

Hello! I'm Shelley, and I have a deep passion for helping individuals of all ages discover the joy of movement in their everyday lives. As I celebrate my 66th year, I am more aware than ever of the adventures that still await us. I invite you to join me on this journey—whether it's on the yoga mat, lifting weights at the gym, or exploring beautiful hiking trails.

I am a Certified Personal Trainer, Kickboxing Instructor, Pilates Instructor, and Group Fitness Leader, equipped with a diverse toolkit to support your fitness journey. Additionally, I hold an RYT 200 certification in yoga, specializing in Yin Yoga, Restorative Yoga, and Trauma-Sensitive Yoga. My mission is to promote a holistic approach to movement that nurtures strength, flexibility, and mindfulness.

Resistance training and yoga have been the cornerstones of my own path to vitality. I find immense joy in honoring my body and spirit through exercise. Beyond my personal lifelong fitness journey, my greatest joy comes from my family. As a proud grandmother to two wonderful granddaughters, Marlowe and Shae, I draw inspiration from life's simplest moments and strive to lead by example.

I can't wait to share this journey of health and happiness with you! Let's embrace movement together—live long, live well, and thrive!

- **Instagram:**
  https://www.instagram.com/murdockshelley/

- **Website:**
  https://fitnesswithshell.com/

- **YouTube:**
  https://www.youtube.com/@shelleymurdock7011

- **LinkedIn:**
  https://www.linkedin.com/in/shelleymurdock/

- **Email:**
  shelleyamurdock@gmail.com

thank you

Thank you for reading my book!

Dear Reader,

Thank you so much for taking the time to read my book! Your support means the world to me, and I genuinely appreciate all your feedback. Hearing your thoughts and experiences is invaluable as I strive to improve my writing and create even better books in the future.

If you found value in this book, I would be incredibly grateful if you could take just two minutes to leave a review on Amazon. Your insights not only help me but also guide other readers on their journey to discovering the best and healthiest version of themselves.

Thank you for choosing this book as a part of your longevity journey. I invite you to follow me on social media, where we can connect and share our longevity habits. Together, we can inspire each other to continue growing and thriving!

Let's embark on this journey together!

With gratitude,

xxoo
Shell

MY GIFT TO YOU

Congratulations on reading this book
and investing in your longevity.

As a special thank you for choosing this book, I'm excited to offer you FREE access to the audiobook of *In Search of Longevity: How to Engineer a Life with Healthy Habits* along with a collection of other valuable resources.

Simply scan the QR code below to claim your gift or visit https://fitnesswithshell.com/

Manufactured by Amazon.ca
Bolton, ON